Ten Days

In a

Mad-House and

Other Stories.

By Nellie Bly

INTRODUCTION.

SINCE my experiences in Blackwell's Island Insane Asylum were published in the *World* I have received hundreds of letters in regard to it. The edition containing my story long since ran out, and I have been prevailed upon to allow it to be published in book form, to satisfy the hundreds who are yet asking for copies.

I am happy to be able to state as a result of my visit to the asylum and the exposures consequent thereon, that the City of New York has appropriated $1,000,000 more per annum than ever before for the care of the insane. So I have at least the satisfaction of knowing that the poor unfortunates will be the better cared for because of my work.

Nellie Bly

TEN DAYS IN A MAD-HOUSE.

CHAPTER I.
A DELICATE MISSION.

ON the 22d of September I was asked by the *World* if I could have myself committed to one of the asylums for the insane in New York, with a view to writing a plain and unvarnished narrative of the treatment of the patients therein and the methods of management, etc. Did I think I had the courage to go through such an ordeal as the mission would demand? Could I assume the characteristics of insanity to such a degree that I could pass the doctors, live for a week among the insane without the authorities there finding out that I was only a "chiel amang 'em takin' notes?" I said I believed I could. I had some faith in my own ability as an actress and thought I could assume insanity long enough to accomplish any mission intrusted to me. Could I pass a week in the insane ward at Blackwell's Island? I said I could and I would. And I did.

My instructions were simply to go on with my work as soon as I felt that I was ready. I was to chronicle faithfully the experiences I underwent, and when once within the walls of the asylum to find out and describe its inside workings, which are always, so effectually hidden by white-capped nurses, as well as by bolts and bars, from the knowledge of the public. "We do not ask you to go there for the purpose of making sensational revelations. Write up things as you find them, good or bad; give praise or blame as you think best, and the truth all the time. But I am afraid of that chronic smile of yours," said the editor. "I will smile no more," I said, and I went away to execute my delicate and, as I found out, difficult mission.

If I did get into the asylum, which I hardly hoped to do, I had no idea that my experiences would contain aught else than a simple tale of life in an asylum. That such an institution could be mismanaged, and that cruelties could exist 'neath its roof, I did not deem possible. I always had a desire to know asylum life more thoroughly–a desire to be convinced that the most helpless of God's creatures, the insane, were cared for kindly and properly. The many stories I had read of abuses in such institutions I had regarded as wildly exaggerated or else romances, yet there was a latent desire to know positively.

I shuddered to think how completely the insane were in the power of their keepers, and how one could weep and plead for release, and all of no avail, if the keepers were so minded. Eagerly I accepted the mission to learn the inside workings of the Blackwell Island Insane Asylum.

"How will you get me out," I asked my editor, "after I once get in?"

"I do not know," he replied, "but we will get you out if we have to tell who you are, and for what purpose you feigned insanity–only get in."

I had little belief in my ability to deceive the insanity experts, and I think my editor had less.

All the preliminary preparations for my ordeal were left to be planned by myself. Only one thing was decided upon, namely, that I should pass under the pseudonym of Nellie Brown, the initials of which would agree with my own name and my linen, so that there would be no difficulty in keeping track of my movements and assisting me out of any difficulties or dangers I might get into. There were ways of getting into the insane ward, but I did not know them. I might adopt one of two courses. Either I could feign insanity at the house of friends, and get myself committed on the decision of two competent physicians, or I could go to my goal by way of the police courts.

NELLIE PRACTICES INSANITY AT HOME.

On reflection I thought it wiser not to inflict myself upon my friends or to get any good-natured doctors to assist me in my purpose. Besides, to get to Blackwell's Island my friends would have had to feign poverty, and, unfortunately for the end I had in view, my acquaintance with the struggling poor, except my own self, was only very superficial. So I determined upon the plan which led me to the successful accomplishment of my mission. I succeeded in getting committed to the insane ward at Blackwell's Island, where I spent ten days and nights and had an experience which I shall never forget. I took upon myself to enact the part of a poor, unfortunate crazy girl, and felt it my duty not to shirk any of the disagreeable results that should follow. I became one of the city's insane wards for that length of time, experienced much, and saw and heard more of the treatment accorded to this helpless class of our population, and when I had seen and heard enough, my release was promptly secured. I left the insane ward with pleasure and regret–pleasure that I was once more able to enjoy the free breath of heaven; regret that I could not have brought with me some of the unfortunate women who lived and suffered with me, and who, I am convinced, are just as sane as I was and am now myself.

But here let me say one thing: From the moment I entered the insane ward on the Island, I made no attempt to keep up the assumed *role* of insanity. I talked and acted just as I do in ordinary life. Yet strange to say, the more sanely I talked and acted the crazier I was thought to be by all except one physician, whose kindness and gentle ways I shall not soon forget.

CHAPTER II.
PREPARING FOR THE ORDEAL.

BUT to return to my work and my mission. After receiving my instructions I returned to my boarding-house, and when evening came I began to practice the *role* in which I was to make my *debut* on the morrow. What a difficult task, I thought, to appear before a crowd of people and convince them that I was insane. I had never been near insane persons before in my life, and had not the faintest idea of what their actions were like. And then to be examined by a number of learned physicians who make insanity a specialty, and who daily come in contact with insane people! How could I hope to pass these doctors and convince them that I was crazy? I feared that they could not be deceived. I began to think my task a hopeless one; but it had to be done. So I flew to the mirror and examined my face. I remembered all I had read of the doings of crazy people, how first of all they have staring eyes, and so I opened mine as wide as possible and stared unblinkingly at my own reflection. I assure you the sight was not reassuring, even to myself, especially in the dead of night. I tried to turn the gas up higher in hopes that it would raise my courage. I succeeded only partially, but I consoled myself with the thought that in a few nights more I would not be there, but locked up in a cell with a lot of lunatics.

The weather was not cold; but, nevertheless, when I thought of what was to come, wintery chills ran races up and down my back in very mockery of the perspiration which was slowly but surely taking the curl out of my bangs. Between times, practicing before the mirror and picturing my future as a lunatic, I read snatches of improbable and impossible ghost stories, so that when the dawn came to chase away the night, I felt that I was in a fit mood for my mission, yet hungry enough to feel keenly that I wanted my breakfast. Slowly and sadly I took my morning bath and quietly bade farewell to a few of the most precious articles known to modern civilization. Tenderly I put my tooth-brush aside, and, when taking a final rub of the soap, I murmured, "It may be for days, and it may be–for longer." Then I donned the old clothing I had selected for the occasion. I was in the mood to look at everything through very serious glasses. It's just as well to take a last "fond look," I mused, for who could tell but that the strain of playing crazy, and being shut up with a crowd of mad people, might turn my own brain, and I would never get back. But not once did I think of shirking my mission. Calmly, outwardly at least, I went out to my crazy business.

I first thought it best to go to a boarding-house, and, after securing lodging, confidentially tell the landlady, or lord, whichever it might chance to be, that I was seeking work, and, in a few days after, apparently go insane. When I reconsidered the idea, I feared it would take too long to mature. Suddenly I thought how much easier it would be to go to a boarding-home for working women. I knew, if once I made a houseful of women believe me crazy, that they would never rest until I was out of their reach and in secure quarters.

From a directory I selected the Temporary Home for Females, No. 84 Second Avenue. As I walked down the avenue, I determined that, once inside the Home, I should do the best I could to get started on my journey to Blackwell's Island and the Insane Asylum.

CHAPTER III.
IN THE TEMPORARY HOME.

I WAS left to begin my career as Nellie Brown, the insane girl. As I walked down the avenue I tried to assume the look which maidens wear in pictures entitled "Dreaming." "Far-away" expressions have a crazy air. I passed through the little paved yard to the entrance of the Home. I pulled the bell, which sounded loud enough for a church chime, and nervously awaited the opening of the door to the Home, which I intended should ere long cast me forth and out upon the charity of the police. The door was thrown back with a vengeance, and a short, yellow-haired girl of some thirteen summers stood before me.

"Is the matron in?" I asked, faintly.

"Yes, she's in; she's busy. Go to the back parlor," answered the girl, in a loud voice, without one change in her peculiarly matured face.

AT THE TEMPORARY HOME FOR WOMEN.

I followed these not overkind or polite instructions and found myself in a dark, uncomfortable back-parlor. There I awaited the arrival of my hostess. I had been seated some twenty minutes at the least, when a slender woman, clad in a plain, dark dress entered and, stopping before me, ejaculated inquiringly, "Well?"

"Are you the matron?" I asked.

"No," she replied, "the matron is sick; I am her assistant. What do you want?"

"I want to stay here for a few days, if you can accommodate me."

"Well, I have no single rooms, we are so crowded; but if you will occupy a room with another girl, I shall do that much for you."

"I shall be glad of that," I answered. "How much do you charge?" I had brought only about seventy cents along with me, knowing full well that the sooner my funds were exhausted the sooner I should be put out, and to be put out was what I was working for.

"We charge thirty cents a night," was her reply to my question, and with that I paid her for one night's lodging, and she left me on the plea of having something else to look after. Left to amuse myself as best I could, I took a survey of my surroundings.

They were not cheerful, to say the least. A wardrobe, desk, book-case, organ, and several chairs completed the furnishment of the room, into which the daylight barely came.

By the time I had become familiar with my quarters a bell, which rivaled the door-bell in its loudness, began clanging in the basement, and simultaneously women went trooping down-stairs from all parts of the house. I imagined, from the obvious signs, that dinner was served, but as no one had said anything to me I made no effort to follow in the hungry train. Yet I did wish that some one would invite me down. It always produces such a lonely, homesick feeling to know others are eating, and we haven't a chance, even if we are not hungry. I was glad when the assistant matron came up and asked me if I did not want something to eat. I replied that I did, and then I asked her what her name was. Mrs. Stanard, she said, and I immediately wrote it down in a notebook I had taken with me for the purpose of making memoranda, and in which I had written several pages of utter nonsense for inquisitive scientists.

Thus equipped I awaited developments. But my dinner—well, I followed Mrs. Stanard down the uncarpeted stairs into the basement; where a large number of women were eating. She found room for me at a table with three other women. The short-haired slavey who had opened the door now put

9

in an appearance as waiter. Placing her arms akimbo and staring me out of countenance she said:

"Boiled mutton, boiled beef, beans, potatoes, coffee or tea?"

"Beef, potatoes, coffee and bread," I responded.

"Bread goes in," she explained, as she made her way to the kitchen, which was in the rear. It was not very long before she returned with what I had ordered on a large, badly battered tray, which she banged down before me. I began my simple meal. It was not very enticing, so while making a feint of eating I watched the others.

I have often moralized on the repulsive form charity always assumes! Here was a home for deserving women and yet what a mockery the name was. The floor was bare, and the little wooden tables were sublimely ignorant of such modern beautifiers as varnish, polish and table-covers. It is useless to talk about the cheapness of linen and its effect on civilization. Yet these honest workers, the most deserving of women, are asked to call this spot of bareness–home.

When the meal was finished each woman went to the desk in the corner, where Mrs. Stanard sat, and paid her bill. I was given a much-used, and abused, red check, by the original piece of humanity in shape of my waitress. My bill was about thirty cents.

After dinner I went up-stairs and resumed my former place in the back parlor. I was quite cold and uncomfortable, and had fully made up my mind that I could not endure that sort of business long, so the sooner I assumed my insane points the sooner I would be released from enforced idleness. Ah! that was indeed the longest day I had ever lived. I listlessly watched the women in the front parlor, where all sat except myself.

One did nothing but read and scratch her head and occasionally call out mildly, "Georgie," without lifting her eyes from her book. "Georgie" was her over-frisky boy, who had more noise in him than any child I ever saw before. He did everything that was rude and unmannerly, I thought, and the mother never said a word unless she heard some one else yell at him. Another woman always kept going to sleep and waking herself up with her own snoring. I really felt wickedly thankful it was only herself she awakened. The majority of the women sat there doing nothing, but there

10

were a few who made lace and knitted unceasingly. The enormous door-bell seemed to be going all the time, and so did the short-haired girl. The latter was, besides, one of those girls who sing all the time snatches of all the songs and hymns that have been composed for the last fifty years. There is such a thing as martyrdom in these days. The ringing of the bell brought more people who wanted shelter for the night. Excepting one woman, who was from the country on a day's shopping expedition, they were working women, some of them with children.

As it drew toward evening Mrs. Stanard came to me and said:

"What is wrong with you? Have you some sorrow or trouble?"

"No," I said, almost stunned at the suggestion. "Why?"

"Oh, because," she said, womanlike, "I can see it in your face. It tells the story of a great trouble."

"Yes, everything is so sad," I said, in a haphazard way, which I had intended to reflect my craziness.

"But you must not allow that to worry you. We all have our troubles, but we get over them in good time. What kind of work are you trying to get?"

"I do not know; it's all so sad," I replied.

"Would you like to be a nurse for children and wear a nice white cap and apron?" she asked.

I put my handkerchief up to my face to hide a smile, and replied in a muffled tone, "I never worked; I don't know how."

"But you must learn," she urged; "all these women here work."

"Do they?" I said, in a low, thrilling whisper. "Why, they look horrible to me; just like crazy women. I am so afraid of them."

"They don't look very nice," she answered, assentingly, "but they are good, honest working women. We do not keep crazy people here."

11

I again used my handkerchief to hide a smile, as I thought that before morning she would at least think she had one crazy person among her flock.

"They all look crazy," I asserted again, "and I am afraid of them. There are so many crazy people about, and one can never tell what they will do. Then there are so many murders committed, and the police never catch the murderers," and I finished with a sob that would have broken up an audience of *blase* critics. She gave a sudden and convulsive start, and I knew my first stroke had gone home. It was amusing to see what a remarkably short time it took her to get up from her chair and to whisper hurriedly: "I'll come back to talk with you after a while." I knew she would not come back and she did not.

When the supper-bell rang I went along with the others to the basement and partook of the evening meal, which was similar to dinner, except that there was a smaller bill of fare and more people, the women who are employed outside during the day having returned. After the evening meal we all adjourned to the parlors, where all sat, or stood, as there were not chairs enough to go round.

It was a wretchedly lonely evening, and the light which fell from the solitary gas jet in the parlor, and oil-lamp the hall, helped to envelop us in a dusky hue and dye our spirits navy blue. I felt it would not require many inundations of this atmosphere to make me a fit subject for the place I was striving to reach.

NELLIE'S FIRST MEAL AT THE HOME.

I watched two women, who seemed of all the crowd to be the most sociable, and I selected them as the ones to work out my salvation, or, more properly speaking, my condemnation and conviction. Excusing myself and saying that I felt lonely, I asked if I might join their company. They graciously consented, so with my hat and gloves on, which no one had asked me to lay aside, I sat down and listened to the rather wearisome conversation, in which I took no part, merely keeping up my sad look, saying "Yes," or "No," or "I can't say," to their observations. Several times I told them I thought everybody in the house looked crazy, but they were slow to catch on to my very original remark. One said her name was Mrs. King and that she was a Southern woman. Then she said that I had a Southern accent. She asked me bluntly if I did not really come from the South. I said "Yes." The other woman got to talking about the Boston boats and asked me if I knew at what time they left.

For a moment I forgot my *role* of assumed insanity, and told her the correct hour of departure. She then asked me what work I was going to do, or if I had ever done any. I replied that I thought it very sad that there were so many working people in the world. She said in reply that she had been unfortunate and had come to New York, where she had worked at correcting proofs on a medical dictionary for some time, but that her health had given way under the task, and that she was now going to Boston again. When the maid came to tell us to go to bed I remarked that I was afraid, and again ventured the assertion that all the women in the house seemed to be crazy. The nurse insisted on my going to bed. I asked if I could not sit on the stairs, but she said, decisively: "No; for every one in the house would think you were crazy." Finally I allowed them to take me to a room.

Here I must introduce a new personage by name into my narrative. It is the woman who had been a proofreader, and was about to return to Boston. She was a Mrs. Caine, who was as courageous as she was good-hearted. She came into my room, and sat and talked with me a long time, taking down my hair with gentle ways. She tried to persuade me to undress and go to bed, but I stubbornly refused to do so. During this time a number of the inmates of the house had gathered around us. They expressed themselves in various ways. "Poor loon!" they said. "Why, she's crazy enough!" "I am afraid to stay with such a crazy being in house." "She will murder us all before morning." One woman was for sending for a policeman to take me at once. They were all in a terrible and real state of fright.

No one wanted to be responsible for me, and the woman who was to occupy the room with me declared that she would not stay with that "crazy woman" for all the money of the Vanderbilts. It was then that Mrs. Caine said she would stay with me. I told her I would like to have her do so. So she was left with me. She didn't undress, but lay down on the bed, watchful of my movements. She tried to induce me to lie down, but I was afraid to do this. I knew that if I once gave way I should fall asleep and dream as pleasantly and peacefully as a child. I should, to use a slang expression, be liable to "give myself dead away." So I insisted on sitting on the side of the bed and staring blankly at vacancy. My poor companion was put into a wretched state of unhappiness. Every few moments she would rise up to look at me. She told me that my eyes shone terribly brightly and then began to question me, asking me where I had lived, how long I had been in New York, what I had been doing, and many things besides. To all her questionings I had but one response–I told her that I had forgotten everything, that ever since my headache had come on I could not remember.

Poor soul! How cruelly I tortured her, and what a kind heart she had! But how I tortured all of them! One of them dreamed of me–as a nightmare. After I had been in the room an hour or so, I was myself startled by hearing a woman screaming in the next room. I began to imagine that I was really in an insane asylum.

Mrs. Caine woke up, looked around, frightened, and listened. She then went out and into the next room, and I heard her asking another woman some questions. When she came back she told me that the woman had had a hideous nightmare. She had been dreaming of me. She had seen me, she said, rushing at her with a knife in my hand, with the intention of killing her. In trying to escape me she had fortunately been able to scream, and so to awaken herself and scare off her nightmare. Then Mrs. Caine got into bed again, considerably agitated, but very sleepy.

I was weary, too, but I had braced myself up to the work, and was determined to keep awake all night so as to carry on my work of impersonation to a successful end in the morning. I heard midnight. I had yet six hours to wait for daylight. The time passed with excruciating slowness. Minutes appeared hours. The noises in the house and on the avenue ceased.

Fearing that sleep would coax me into its grasp, I commenced to review my life. How strange it all seems! One incident, if never so trifling, is but a link more to chain us to our unchangeable fate. I began at the beginning,

14

and lived again the story of my life. Old friends were recalled with a pleasurable thrill; old enmities, old heartaches, old joys were once again present. The turned-down pages of my life were turned up, and the past was present.

When it was completed, I turned my thoughts bravely to the future, wondering, first, what the next day would bring forth, then making plans for the carrying out of my project. I wondered if I should be able to pass over the river to the goal of my strange ambition, to become eventually an inmate of the halls inhabited by my mentally wrecked sisters. And then, once in, what would be my experience? And after? How to get out? Bah! I said, they will get me out.

That was the greatest night of my existence. For a few hours I stood face to face with "self!"

I looked out toward the window and hailed with joy the slight shimmer of dawn. The light grew strong and gray, but the silence was strikingly still. My companion slept. I had still an hour or two to pass over. Fortunately I found some employment for my mental activity. Robert Bruce in his captivity had won confidence in the future, and passed his time as pleasantly as possible under the circumstances, by watching the celebrated spider building his web. I had less noble vermin to interest me. Yet I believe I made some valuable discoveries in natural history. I was about to drop off to sleep in spite of myself when I was suddenly startled to wakefulness. I thought I heard something crawl and fall down upon the counterpane with an almost inaudible thud.

I had the opportunity of studying these interesting animals very thoroughly. They had evidently come for breakfast, and were not a little disappointed to find that their principal *plat* was not there. They scampered up and down the pillow, came together, seemed to hold interesting converse, and acted in every way as if they were puzzled by the absence of an appetizing breakfast. After one consultation of some length they finally disappeared, seeking victims elsewhere, and leaving me to pass the long minutes by giving my attention to cockroaches, whose size and agility were something of a surprise to me.

My room companion had been sound asleep for a long time, but she now woke up, and expressed surprise at seeing me still awake and apparently as lively as a cricket. She was as sympathetic as ever. She came to me and took my hands and tried her best to console me, and asked me if I did not want to go home. She kept me up-stairs until nearly everybody was out of the house, and then took me down to the basement for coffee and a bun. After that, partaken in silence, I went back to my room, where I sat down, moping. Mrs. Caine grew more and more anxious. "What is to be done?" she kept exclaiming. "Where are your friends?" "No," I answered, "I have no friends, but I have some trunks. Where are they? I want them." The good woman tried to pacify me, saying that they would be found in good time. She believed that I was insane.

Yet I forgive her. It is only after one is in trouble that one realizes how little sympathy and kindness there are in the world. The women in the Home who were not afraid of me had wanted to have some amusement at my expense, and so they had bothered me with questions and remarks that had I been insane would have been cruel and inhumane. Only this one woman among the crowd, pretty and delicate Mrs. Caine, displayed true womanly feeling. She compelled the others to cease teasing me and took the bed of the woman who refused to sleep near me. She protested against the suggestion to leave me alone and to have me locked up for the night so that I could harm no one. She insisted on remaining with me in order to administer aid should I need it. She smoothed my hair and bathed my brow and talked as soothingly to me as a mother would do to an ailing child. By every means she tried to have me go to bed and rest, and when it drew toward morning she got up and wrapped a blanket around me for fear I might get cold; then she kissed me on the brow and whispered, compassionately:

"Poor child, poor child!"

How much I admired that little woman's courage and kindness. How I longed to reassure her and whisper that I was not insane, and how I hoped that, if any poor girl should ever be so unfortunate as to be what I was pretending to be, she might meet with one who possessed the same spirit of human kindness possessed by Mrs. Ruth Caine.

CHAPTER IV.
JUDGE DUFFY AND THE POLICE.

BUT to return to my story. I kept up my *role* until the assistant matron, Mrs. Stanard, came in. She tried to persuade me to be calm. I began to see clearly that she wanted to get me out of the house at all hazards, quietly if possible. This I did not want. I refused to move, but kept up ever the refrain of my lost trunks. Finally some one suggested that an officer be sent for. After awhile Mrs. Stanard put on her bonnet and went out. Then I knew that I was making an advance toward the home of the insane. Soon she returned, bringing with her two policemen–big, strong men–who entered the room rather unceremoniously, evidently expecting to meet with a person violently crazy. The name of one of them was Tom Bockert.

When they entered I pretended not to see them. "I want you to take her quietly," said Mrs. Stanard. "If she don't come along quietly," responded one of the men, "I will drag her through the streets." I still took no notice of them, but certainly wished to avoid raising a scandal outside. Fortunately Mrs. Caine came to my rescue. She told the officers about my outcries for my lost trunks, and together they made up a plan to get me to go along with them quietly by telling me they would go with me to look for my lost effects. They asked me if I would go. I said I was afraid to go alone. Mrs. Stanard then said she would accompany me, and she arranged that the two policemen should follow us at a respectful distance. She tied on my veil for me, and we left the house by the basement and started across town, the two officers following at some distance behind. We walked along very quietly and finally came to the station house, which the good woman assured me was the express office, and that there we should certainly find my missing effects. I went inside with fear and trembling, for good reason.

A few days previous to this I had met Captain McCullagh at a meeting held in Cooper Union. At that time I had asked him for some information which he had given me. If he were in, would he not recognize me? And then all would be lost so far as getting to the island was concerned. I pulled my sailor hat as low down over my face as I possibly could, and prepared for the ordeal. Sure enough there was sturdy Captain McCullagh standing near the desk.

He watched me closely as the officer at the desk conversed in a low tone with Mrs. Stanard and the policeman who brought me.

"Are you Nellie Brown?" asked the officer. I said I supposed I was. "Where do you come from?" he asked. I told him I did not know, and then Mrs. Stanard gave him a lot of information about me–told him how strangely I had acted at her home; how I had not slept a wink all night, and that in her opinion I was a poor unfortunate who had been driven crazy by inhuman treatment. There was some discussion between Mrs. Standard and the two officers, and Tom Bockert was told to take us down to the court in a car.

IN THE HANDS OF THE POLICE.

"Come along," Bockert said, "I will find your trunk for you." We all went together, Mrs. Stanard, Tom Bockert, and myself. I said it was very kind of them to go with me, and I should not soon forget them. As we walked along I kept up my refrain about my trucks, injecting occasionally some remark about the dirty condition of the streets and the curious character of the people we met on the way. "I don't think I have ever seen such people before," I said. "Who are they?" I asked, and my companions looked upon me with expressions of pity, evidently believing I was a foreigner, an emigrant or something of the sort. They told me that the people around me were working people. I remarked once more that I thought there were too many working people in the world for the amount of work to be done, at which remark Policeman P. T. Bockert eyed me closely, evidently thinking that my mind was gone for good. We passed several other policemen, who generally asked my sturdy guardians what was the matter with me. By this time quite a number of ragged children were following us too, and they passed remarks about me that were to me original as well as amusing.

"What's she up for?" "Say, kop, where did ye get her?" "Where did yer pull 'er?" "She's a daisy!"

Poor Mrs. Stanard was more frightened than I was. The whole situation grew interesting, but I still had fears for my fate before the judge.

At last we came to a low building, and Tom Bockert kindly volunteered the information: "Here's the express office. We shall soon find those trunks of yours."

The entrance to the building was surrounded by a curious crowd and I did not think my case was bad enough to permit me passing them without some remark, so I asked if all those people had lost their trunks.

"Yes," he said, "nearly all these people are looking for trunks."

I said, "They all seem to be foreigners, too." "Yes," said Tom, "they are all foreigners just landed. They have all lost their trunks, and it takes most of our time to help find them for them."

We entered the courtroom. It was the Essex Market Police Courtroom. At last the question of my sanity or insanity was to be decided. Judge Duffy sat behind the high desk, wearing a look which seemed to indicate that he was dealing out the milk of human kindness by wholesale. I rather feared I would not get the fate I sought, because of the kindness I saw on every line of his face, and it was with rather a sinking heart that I followed Mrs. Stanard as she answered the summons to go up to the desk, where Tom Bockert had just given an account of the affair.

"Come here," said an officer. "What is your name?"

"Nellie Brown," I replied, with a little accent. "I have lost my trunks, and would like if you could find them."

"When did you come to New York?" he asked.

"I did not come to New York," I replied (while I added, mentally, "because I have been here for some time.")

"But you are in New York now," said the man.

"No," I said, looking as incredulous as I thought a crazy person could, "I did not come to New York."

19

"That girl is from the west," he said, in a tone that made me tremble. "She has a western accent."

Some one else who had been listening to the brief dialogue here asserted that he had lived south and that my accent was southern, while another officer was positive it was eastern. I felt much relieved when the first spokesman turned to the judge and said:

"Judge, here is a peculiar case of a young woman who doesn't know who she is or where she came from. You had better attend to it at once."

I commenced to shake with more than the cold, and I looked around at the strange crowd about me, composed of poorly dressed men and women with stories printed on their faces of hard lives, abuse and poverty. Some were consulting eagerly with friends, while others sat still with a look of utter hopelessness. Everywhere was a sprinkling of well-dressed, well-fed officers watching the scene passively and almost indifferently. It was only an old story with them. One more unfortunate added to a long list which had long since ceased to be of any interest or concern to them.

NELLIE BEFORE JUDGE DUFFY.

"Come here, girl, and lift your veil," called out Judge Duffy, in tones which surprised me by a harshness which I did not think from the kindly face he possessed.

"Who are you speaking to?" I inquired, in my stateliest manner.

20

"Come here, my dear, and lift your veil. You know the Queen of England, if she were here, would have to lift her veil," he said, very kindly.

"That is much better," I replied. "I am not the Queen of England, but I'll lift my veil."

As I did so the little judge looked at me, and then, in a very kind and gentle tone, he said:

"My dear child, what is wrong?"

"Nothing is wrong except that I have lost my trunks, and this man," indicating Policeman Bockert, "promised to bring me where they could be found."

"What do you know about this child?" asked the judge, sternly, of Mrs. Stanard, who stood, pale and trembling, by my side.

"I know nothing of her except that she came to the home yesterday and asked to remain overnight."

"The home! What do you mean by the home?" asked Judge Duffy, quickly.

"It is a temporary home kept for working women at No. 84 Second Avenue."

"What is your position there?"

"I am assistant matron."

"Well, tell us all you know of the case."

"When I was going into the home yesterday I noticed her coming down the avenue. She was all alone. I had just got into the house when the bell rang and she came in. When I talked with her she wanted to know if she could stay all night, and I said she could. After awhile she said all the people in the house looked crazy, and she was afraid of them. Then she would not go to bed, but sat up all the night."

"Had she any money?"

"Yes," I replied, answering for her, "I paid her for everything, and the eating was the worst I ever tried."

There was a general smile at this, and some murmurs of "She's not so crazy on the food question."

"Poor child," said Judge Duffy, "she is well dressed, and a lady. Her English is perfect, and I would stake everything on her being a good girl. I am positive she is somebody's darling."

At this announcement everybody laughed, and I put my handkerchief over my face and endeavored to choke the laughter that threatened to spoil my plans, in despite of my resolutions.

"I mean she is some woman's darling," hastily amended the judge. "I am sure some one is searching for her. Poor girl, I will be good to her, for she looks like my sister, who is dead."

There was a hush for a moment after this announcement, and the officers glanced at me more kindly, while I silently blessed the kind-hearted judge, and hoped that any poor creatures who might be afflicted as I pretended to be should have as kindly a man to deal with as Judge Duffy.

"I wish the reporters were here," he said at last. "They would be able to find out something about her."

I got very much frightened at this, for if there is any one who can ferret out a mystery it is a reporter. I felt that I would rather face a mass of expert doctors, policemen, and detectives than two bright specimens of my craft, so I said:

"I don't see why all this is needed to help me find my trunks. These men are impudent, and I do not want to be stared at. I will go away. I don't want to stay here."

So saying, I pulled down my veil and secretly hoped the reporters would be detained elsewhere until I was sent to the asylum.

"I don't know what to do with the poor child," said the worried judge. "She must be taken care of."

"Send her to the Island," suggested one of the officers.

"Oh, don't!" said Mrs. Stanard, in evident alarm. "Don't! She is a lady and it would kill her to be put on the Island."

For once I felt like shaking the good woman. To think the Island was just the place I wanted to reach and here she was trying to keep me from going there! It was very kind of her, but rather provoking under the circumstances.

"There has been some foul work here," said the judge. "I believe this child has been drugged and brought to this city. Make out the papers and we will send her to Bellevue for examination. Probably in a few days the effect of the drug will pass off and she will be able to tell us a story that will be startling. If the reporters would only come!"

I dreaded them, so I said something about not wishing to stay there any longer to be gazed at. Judge Duffy then told Policeman Bockert to take me to the back office. After we were seated there Judge Duffy came in and asked me if my home was in Cuba.

"Yes," I replied, with a smile. "How did you know?"

"Oh, I knew it, my dear. Now, tell me were was it? In what part of Cuba?"

"On the hacienda," I replied.

"Ah," said the judge, "on a farm. Do you remember Havana?"

"Si, senor," I answered; "it is near home. How did you know?"

"Oh, I knew all about it. Now, won't you tell me the name of your home?" he asked, persuasively.

"That's what I forget," I answered, sadly. "I have a headache all the time, and it makes me forget things. I don't want them to trouble me. Everybody is asking me questions, and it makes my head worse," and in truth it did.

"Well, no one shall trouble you any more. Sit down here and rest awhile," and the genial judge left me alone with Mrs. Stanard.

23

Just then an officer came in with a reporter. I was so frightened, and thought I would be recognized as a journalist, so I turned my head away and said, "I don't want to see any reporters; I will not see any; the judge said I was not to be troubled."

"Well, there is no insanity in that," said the man who had brought the reporter, and together they left the room. Once again I had a fit of fear. Had I gone too far in not wanting to see a reporter, and was my sanity detected? If I had given the impression that I was sane, I was determined to undo it, so I jumped up and ran back and forward through the office, Mrs. Stanard clinging terrified to my arm.

"I won't stay here; I want my trunks! Why do they bother me with so many people?" and thus I kept on until the ambulance surgeon came in, accompanied by the judge.

CHAPTER V.
PRONOUNCED INSANE.

"HERE is a poor girl who has been drugged," explained the judge. "She looks like my sister, and any one can see she is a good girl. I am interested in the child, and I would do as much for her as if she were my own. I want you to be kind to her," he said to the ambulance surgeon. Then, turning to Mrs. Stanard, he asked her if she could not keep me for a few days until my case was inquired into. Fortunately, she said she could not, because all the women at the Home were afraid of me, and would leave if I were kept there. I was very much afraid she would keep me if the pay was assured her, and so I said something about the bad cooking and that I did not intend to go back to the Home. Then came the examination; the doctor looked clever and I had not one hope of deceiving him, but I determined to keep up the farce.

"Put out your tongue," he ordered, briskly.

I gave an inward chuckle at the thought.

"Put out your tongue when I tell you," he said.

"I don't want to," I answered, truthfully enough.

"You must. You are sick, and I am a doctor."

"I am not sick and never was. I only want my trunks."

But I put out my tongue, which he looked at in a sagacious manner. Then he felt my pulse and listened to the beating of my heart. I had not the least idea how the heart of an insane person beat, so I held my breath all the while he listened, until, when he quit, I had to give a gasp to regain it. Then he tried the effect of the light on the pupils of my eyes. Holding his hand within a half inch of my face, he told me to look at it, then, jerking it hastily away, he would examine my eyes. I was puzzled to know what insanity was like in the eye, so I thought the best thing under the circumstances was to stare. This I did. I held my eyes riveted unblinkingly upon his hand, and when he removed it I exerted all my strength to still keep my eyes from blinking.

AN INSANITY EXPERT AT WORK.

"What drugs have you been taking?" he then asked me.

"Drugs!" I repeated, wonderingly. "I do not know what drugs are."

"The pupils of her eyes have been enlarged ever since she came to the Home. They have not changed once," explained Mrs. Stanard. I wondered how she knew whether they had or not, but I kept quiet.

"I believe she has been using belladonna," said the doctor, and for the first time I was thankful that I was a little near-sighted, which of course answers for the enlargement of the pupils. I thought I might as well be truthful when I could without injuring my case, so I told him I was near-sighted, that I was not in the least ill, had never been sick, and that no one had a right to detain me when I wanted to find my trunks. I wanted to go home. He wrote a lot of things in a long, slender book, and then said he was going to take me home. The judge told him to take me and to be kind to me, and to tell the people at the hospital to be kind to me, and to do all they could for me. If we only had more such men as Judge Duffy, the poor unfortunates would not find life all darkness.

I began to have more confidence in my own ability now, since one judge, one doctor, and a mass of people had pronounced me insane, and I put on my veil quite gladly when I was told that I was to be taken in a carriage, and that afterward I could go home. "I am so glad to go with you," I said, and I meant it. I was very glad indeed. Once more, guarded by Policeman Brockert, I walked through the little, crowded courtroom. I felt quite proud of myself as I went out a side door into an alleyway, where the ambulance was waiting. Near the closed and barred gates was a small office occupied by several men and large books. We all went in there, and when they began to ask me questions the doctor interposed and said he had all the papers, and that it was useless to ask me anything further, because I was unable to answer questions. This was a great relief to me, for my nerves were already feeling the strain. A rough-looking man wanted to put me into the ambulance, but I refused his aid so decidedly that the doctor and policeman told him to desist, and they performed that gallant office themselves. I did not enter the ambulance without protest. I made the remark that I had never seen a carriage of that make before, and that I did not want to ride in it, but after awhile I let them persuade me, as I had right along intended to do.

I shall never forget that ride. After I was put in flat on the yellow blanket, the doctor got in and sat near the door. The large gates were swung open, and the curious crowd which had collected swayed back to make way for the ambulance as it backed out. How they tried to get a glimpse at the supposed crazy girl! The doctor saw that I did not like the people gazing at me, and considerately put down the curtains, after asking my wishes in regard to it. Still that did not keep the people away. The children raced after us, yelling all sorts of slang expressions, and trying to get a peep under the curtains. It was quite an interesting drive, but I must say that it was an excruciatingly rough one. I held on, only there was not much to hold on to, and the driver drove as if he feared some one would catch up with us.

CHAPTER VI.
IN BELLEVUE HOSPITAL.

AT last Bellevue was reached, the third station on my way to the island. I had passed through successfully the ordeals at the home and at Essex Market Police Court, and now felt confident that I should not fail. The ambulance stopped with a sudden jerk and the doctor jumped out. "How many have you?" I heard some one inquire. "Only one, for the pavilion," was the reply. A rough-looking man came forward, and catching hold of me attempted to drag me out as if I had the strength of an elephant and would resist. The doctor, seeing my look of disgust, ordered him to leave me alone, saying that he would take charge of me himself. He then lifted me carefully out and I walked with the grace of a queen past the crowd that had gathered curious to see the new unfortunate. Together with the doctor I entered a small dark office, where there were several men. The one behind the desk opened a book and began on the long string of questions which had been asked me so often.

I refused to answer, and the doctor told him it was not necessary to trouble me further, as he had all the papers made out, and I was too insane to be able to tell anything that would be of consequence. I felt relieved that it was so easy here, as, though still undaunted, I had begun to feel faint for want of food. The order was then given to take me to the insane pavilion, and a muscular man came forward and caught me so tightly by the arm that a pain ran clear through me. It made me angry, and for a moment I forgot my *role* as I turned to him and said:

"How dare you touch me?" At this he loosened his hold somewhat, and I shook him off with more strength than I thought I possessed.

"I will go with no one but this man," I said, pointing to the ambulance-surgeon. "The judge said that he was to take care of me, and I will go with no one else."

At this the surgeon said that he would take me, and so we went arm in arm, following the man who had at first been so rough with me. We passed through the well-cared-for grounds and finally reached the insane ward. A white-capped nurse was there to receive me.

"This young girl is to wait here for the boat," said the surgeon, and then he started to leave me. I begged him not to go, or to take me with him, but he said he wanted to get his dinner first, and that I should wait there for him. When I insisted on accompanying him he claimed that he had to assist at an amputation, and it would not look well for me to be present. It was evident that he believed he was dealing with an insane person. Just then the most horrible insane cries came from a yard in the rear. With all my bravery I felt a chill at the prospect of being shut up with a fellow-creature who was really insane. The doctor evidently noticed my nervousness, for he said to the attendant;

"What a noise the carpenters make."

Turning to me he offered me explanation to the effect that new buildings were being erected, and that the noise came from some of the workmen engaged upon it. I told him I did not want to stay there without him, and to pacify me he promised soon to return. He left me and I found myself at last an occupant of an insane asylum.

I stood at the door and contemplated the scene before me. The long, uncarpeted hall was scrubbed to that peculiar whiteness seen only in public institutions. In the rear of the hall were large iron doors fastened by a padlock. Several still-looking benches and a number of willow chairs were the only articles of furniture. On either side of the hall were doors leading into what I supposed and what proved to be bedrooms. Near the entrance door, on the right-hand side, was a small sitting-room for the nurses, and opposite it was a room where dinner was dished out. A nurse in a black dress, white cap and apron and armed with a bunch of keys had charge of the hall. I soon learned her name, Miss Ball.

An old Irishwoman was maid-of-all-work. I heard her called Mary, and I am glad to know that there is such a good-hearted woman in that place. I experienced only kindness and the utmost consideration from her. There were only three patients, as they are called. I made the fourth. I thought I might as well begin work at once, for I still expected that the very first doctor might declare me sane and send me out again into the wide, wide world. So I went down to the rear of the room and introduced myself to one of the women, and asked her all about herself. Her name, she said, was Miss Anne Neville, and she had been sick from overwork. She had been working as a chambermaid, and when her health gave way she was sent to some Sisters' Home to be treated. Her nephew, who was a waiter, was out of work, and, being unable to pay her expenses at the Home, had had her transferred to Bellevue.

"Is there anything wrong with you mentally as well?" I asked her.

"No," she said. "The doctors have been asking me many curious questions and confusing me as much as possible, but I have nothing wrong with my brain."

"Do you know that only insane people are sent to this pavilion?" I asked.

"Yes, I know; but I am unable to do anything. The doctors refuse to listen to me, and it is useless to say anything to the nurses."

Satisfied from various reasons that Miss Neville was as sane as I was myself, I transferred my attentions to one of the other patients. I found her in need of medical aid and quite silly mentally, although I have seen many women in the lower walks of life, whose sanity was never questioned, who were not any brighter.

The third patient, Mrs. Fox, would not say much. She was very quiet, and after telling me that her case was hopeless refused to talk. I began now to feel surer of my position, and I determined that no doctor should convince me that I was sane so long as I had the hope of accomplishing my mission. A small, fair-complexioned nurse arrived, and, after putting on her cap, told Miss Ball to go to dinner. The new nurse, Miss Scott by name, came to me and said, rudely:

"Take off your hat."

"I shall not take off my hat," I answered. "I am waiting for the boat, and I shall not remove it."

"Well, you are not going on any boat. You might as well know it now as later. You are in an asylum for the insane."

Although fully aware of that fact, her unvarnished words gave me a shock. "I did not want to come here; I am not sick or insane, and I will not stay," I said.

30

"It will be a long time before you get out if you don't do as you are told," answered Miss Scott. "You might as well take off your hat, or I shall use force, and if I am not able to do it, I have but to touch a bell and I shall get assistance. Will you take it off?"

"No, I will not. I am cold, and I want my hat on, and you can't make me take it off."

"I shall give you a few more minutes, and if you don't take it off then I shall use force, and I warn you it will not be very gentle."

"If you take my hat off I shall take your cap off; so now."

Miss Scott was called to the door then, and as I feared that an exhibition of temper might show too much sanity I took off my hat and gloves and was sitting quietly looking into space when she returned. I was hungry, and was quite pleased to see Mary make preparations for dinner. The preparations were simple. She merely pulled a straight bench up along the side of a bare table and ordered the patients to gather 'round the feast; then she brought out a small tin plate on which was a piece of boiled meat and a potato. It could not have been colder had it been cooked the week before, and it had no chance to make acquaintance with salt or pepper. I would not go up to the table, so Mary came to where I sat in a corner, and while handing out the tin plate, asked:

"Have ye any pennies about ye, dearie?"

"What?" I said, in my surprise.

"Have ye any pennies, dearie, that ye could give me. They'll take them all from ye any way, dearie, so I might as well have them."

I understood it fully now, but I had no intention of feeing Mary so early in the game, fearing it would have an influence on her treatment of me, so I said I had lost my purse, which was quite true. But though I did not give Mary any money, she was none the less kind to me. When I objected to the tin plate in which she had brought my food she fetched a china one for me, and when I found it impossible to eat the food she presented she gave me a glass of milk and a soda cracker.

All the windows in the hall were open and the cold air began to tell on my Southern blood. It grew so cold indeed as to be almost unbearable, and I complained of it to Miss Scott and Miss Ball. But they answered curtly that as I was in a charity place I could not expect much else. All the other women were suffering from the cold, and the nurses themselves had to wear heavy garments to keep themselves warm. I asked if I could go to bed. They said "No!" At last Miss Scott got an old gray shawl, and shaking some of the moths out of it, told me to put it on.

"It's rather a bad-looking shawl," I said.

"Well, some people would get along better if they were not so proud," said Miss Scott. "People on charity should not expect anything and should not complain."

So I put the moth-eaten shawl, with all its musty smell, around me, and sat down on a wicker chair, wondering what would come next, whether I should freeze to death or survive. My nose was very cold, so I covered up my head and was in a half doze, when the shawl was suddenly jerked from my face and a strange man and Miss Scott stood before me. The man proved to be a doctor, and his first greetings were:

"I've seen that face before."

"Then you know me?" I asked, with a great show of eagerness that I did not feel.

"I think I do. Where did you come from?"

"From home."

"Where is home?"

"Don't you know? Cuba."

POSITIVELY DEMENTED.

He then sat down beside me, felt my pulse, and examined my tongue, and at last said:

"Tell Miss Scott all about yourself."

"No, I will not. I will not talk with women."

"What do you do in New York?"

"Nothing."

"Can you work?"

"No, senor."

"Tell me, are you a woman of the town?"

"I do not understand you," I replied, heartily disgusted with him.

"I mean have you allowed the men to provide for you and keep you?"

I felt like slapping him in the face, but I had to maintain my composure, so I simply said:

"I do not know what you are talking about. I always lived at home."

After many more questions, fully as useless and senseless, he left me and began to talk with the nurse. "Positively demented," he said. "I consider it a hopeless case. She needs to be put where some one will take care of her."

And so I passed my second medical expert.

After this, I began to have a smaller regard for the ability of doctors than I ever had before, and a greater one for myself. I felt sure now that no doctor could tell whether people were insane or not, so long as the case was not violent.

Later in the afternoon a boy and a woman came. The woman sat down on a bench, while the boy went in and talked with Miss Scott. In a short time he came out, and, just nodding good-bye to the woman, who was his mother, went away. She did not look insane, but as she was German I could not learn her story. Her name, however, was Mrs. Louise Schanz. She seemed quite lost, but when the nurses put her at some sewing she did her work well and quickly. At three in the afternoon all the patients were given a gruel broth, and at five a cup of tea and a piece of bread. I was favored; for when they saw that it was impossible for me to eat the bread or drink the stuff honored by the name of tea, they gave me a cup of milk and a cracker, the same as I had had at noon.

Just as the gas was being lighted another patient was added. She was a young girl, twenty-five years old. She told me that she had just gotten up from a sick bed. Her appearance confirmed her story. She looked like one who had had a severe attack of fever. "I am now suffering from nervous debility," she said, "and my friends have sent me here to be treated for it." I did not tell her where she was, and she seemed quite satisfied. At 6.15 Miss Ball said that she wanted to go away, and so we would all have to go to bed. Then each of us—we now numbered six—were assigned a room and told to undress. I did so, and was given a short, cotton-flannel gown to wear during the night. Then she took every particle of the clothing I had worn during the day, and, making it up in a bundle, labeled it "Brown," and took it away. The iron-barred window was locked, and Miss Ball, after giving me an extra blanket, which, she said, was a favor rarely granted, went out and left me alone. The bed was not a comfortable one. It was so hard, indeed, that I could not make a dent in it; and the pillow was stuffed with straw. Under the sheet was an oilcloth spread. As the night grew colder I tried to warm that oilcloth. I kept on trying, but when morning dawned and it was still as cold as when I went to bed, and had reduced me too, to the temperature of an iceberg, I gave it up as an impossible task.

I had hoped to get some rest on this my first night in an insane asylum. But I was doomed to disappointment. When the night nurses came in they were curious to see me and to find out what I was like. No sooner had they left than I heard some one at my door inquiring for Nellie Brown, and I began to tremble, fearing always that my sanity would be discovered. By listening to the conversation I found it was a reporter in search of me, and I heard him ask for my clothing so that he might examine it. I listened quite anxiously to the talk about me, and was relieved to learn that I was considered hopelessly insane. That was encouraging. After the reporter left I heard new arrivals, and I learned that a doctor was there and intended to see me. For what purpose I knew not, and I imagined all sorts of horrible things, such as examinations and the rest of it, and when they got to my room I was shaking with more than fear.

"Nellie Brown, here is the doctor; he wishes to speak with you," said the nurse. If that's all he wanted I thought I could endure it. I removed the blanket which I had put over my head in my sudden fright and looked up. The sight was reassuring.

He was a handsome young man. He had the air and address of a gentleman. Some people have since censured this action; but I feel sure, even if it was a little indiscreet, that they young doctor only meant kindness to me. He came forward, seated himself on the side of my bed, and put his arm soothingly around my shoulders. It was a terrible task to play insane before this young man, and only a girl can sympathize with me in my position.

"How do you feel to-night, Nellie?" he asked, easily.

"Oh, I feel all right."

"But you are sick, you know," he said.

"Oh, am I?" I replied, and I turned by head on the pillow and smiled.

"When did you leave Cuba, Nellie?"

"Oh, you know my home?" I asked.

"Yes, very well. Don't you remember me? I remember you."

"Do you?" and I mentally said I should not forget him. He was accompanied by a friend who never ventured a remark, but stood staring at me as I lay in bed. After a great many questions, to which I answered truthfully, he left me. Then came other troubles. All night long the nurses read one to the other aloud, and I know that the other patients, as well as myself, were unable to sleep. Every half-hour or hour they would walk heavily down the halls, their boot-heels resounding like the march of a private of dragoons, and take a look at every patient. Of course this helped to keep us awake. Then as it came toward morning, they began to beat eggs for breakfast, and the sound made me realize how horribly hungry I was. Occasional yells and cries came from the male department, and that did not aid in making the night pass more cheerfully. Then the ambulance-gong, as it brought in more unfortunates, sounded as a knell to life and liberty. Thus I passed my first night as an insane girl at Bellevue.

CHAPTER VII.
THE GOAL IN SIGHT.

AT 6 o'clock on Sunday morning, Sept. 25, the nurses pulled the covering from my bed. "Come, it's time for you to get out of bed," they said, and opened the window and let in the cold breeze. My clothing was then returned to me. After dressing I was shown to a washstand, where all the other patients were trying to rid their faces of all traces of sleep. At 7 o'clock we were given some horrible mess, which Mary told us was chicken broth. The cold, from which we had suffered enough the day previous, was bitter, and when I complained to the nurse she said it was one of the rules of the institution not to turn the heat on until October, and so we would have to endure it, as the steam-pipes had not even been put in order. The night nurses then, arming themselves with scissors, began to play manicure on the patients. They cut my nails to the quick, as they did those of several of the other patients. Shortly after this a handsome young doctor made his appearance and I was conducted into the sitting-room.

"Who are you?" he asked.

"Nellie Moreno," I replied.

"Then why did you give the name of Brown?" he asked. "What is wrong with you?"

"Nothing. I did not want to come here, but they brought me. I want to go away. Won't you let me out?"

"If I take you out will you stay with me? Won't you run away from me when you get on the street?"

"I can't promise that I will not," I answered, with a smile and a sigh, for he was handsome.

He asked me many other questions. Did I ever see faces on the wall? Did I ever hear voices around? I answered him to the best of my ability.

"Do you ever hear voices at night?" he asked.

"Yes, there is so much talking I cannot sleep."

"I thought so," he said to himself. Then turning to me, he asked: "What do these voices say?"

"Well, I do not listen to them always. But sometimes, very often, they talk about Nellie Brown, and then on other subjects that do not interest me half so much," I answered, truthfully.

"That will do," he said to Miss Scott, who was just on the outside.

"Can I go away?" I asked.

"Yes," he said, with a satisfied laugh, "we'll soon send you away."

"It is so very cold here, I want to go out," I said.

"That's true," he said to Miss Scott. "The cold is almost unbearable in here, and you will have some cases of pneumonia if you are not careful."

With this I was led away and another patient was taken in. I sat right outside the door and waited to hear how he would test the sanity of the other patients. With little variation the examination was exactly the same as mine. All the patients were asked if they saw faces on the wall, heard voices, and what they said. I might also add each patient denied any such peculiar freaks of sight and hearing. At 10 o'clock we were given a cup of unsalted beef tea; at noon a bit of cold meat and a potatoe, at 3 o'clock a cup of oatmeal gruel and at 5.30 a cup of tea and a slice of unbuttered bread. We were all cold and hungry. After the physician left we were given shawls and told to walk up and down the halls in order to get warm. During the day the pavilion was visited by a number of people who were curious to see the crazy girl from Cuba. I kept my head covered, on the plea of being cold, for fear some of the reporters would recognize me. Some of the visitors were apparently in search of a missing girl, for I was made take down the shawl repeatedly, and after they looked at me they would say, "I don't know her," "or [sic], "she is not the one," for which I was secretly thankful. Warden O'Rourke visited me, and tried his arts on an examination. Then he brought some well-dressed women and some gentlemen at different times to have a glance at the mysterious Nellie Brown.

The reporters were the most troublesome. Such a number of them! And they were all so bright and clever that I was terribly frightened lest they

38

should see that I was sane. They were very kind and nice to me, and very gentle in all their questionings. My late visitor the night previous came to the window while some reporters were interviewing me in the sitting-room, and told the nurse to allow them to see me, as they would be of assistance in finding some clew as to my identity.

In the afternoon Dr. Field came and examined me. He asked me only a few questions, and one that had no bearing on such a case. The chief question was of my home and friends, and if I had any lovers or had ever been married. Then he made me stretch out my arms and move my fingers, which I did without the least hesitation, yet I heard him say my case was hopeless. The other patients were asked the same questions.

As the doctor was about to leave the pavilion Miss Tillie Mayard discovered that she was in an insane ward. She went to Dr. Field and asked him why she had been sent there.

"Have you just found out you are in an insane asylum?" asked the doctor.

"Yes; my friends said they were sending me to a convalescent ward to be treated for nervous debility, from which I am suffering since my illness. I want to get out of this place immediately."

"Well, you won't get out in a hurry," he said, with a quick laugh.

"If you know anything at all," she responded, "you should be able to tell that I am perfectly sane. Why don't you test me?"

"We know all we want to on that score," said the doctor, and he left the poor girl condemned to an insane asylum, probably for life, without giving her one feeble chance to prove her sanity.

Sunday night was but a repetition of Saturday. All night long we were kept awake by the talk of the nurses and their heavy walking through the uncarpeted halls. On Monday morning we were told that we should be taken away at 1.30. The nurses questioned me unceasingly about my home, and all seemed to have an idea that I had a lover who had cast me forth on the world and wrecked my brain. The morning brought many reporters. How untiring they are in their efforts to get something new. Miss Scott refused to allow me to be seen, however, and for this I was thankful. Had they been given free access to me, I should probably not have been a

39

mystery long, for many of them knew me by sight. Warden O'Rourke came for a final visit and had a short conversation with me. He wrote his name in my notebook, saying to the nurse that I would forget all about it in an hour. I smiled and thought I wasn't sure of that. Other people called to see me, but none knew me or could give any information about me.

Noon came. I grew nervous as the time approached to leave for the Island. I dreaded every new arrival, fearful that my secret would be discovered at the last moment. Then I was given a shawl and my hat and gloves. I could hardly put them on, my nerves were so unstrung. At last the attendant arrived, and I bade good-bye to Mary as I slipped "a few pennies" into her hand. "God bless you," she said; "I shall pray for you. Cheer up, dearie. You are young, and will get over this." I told her I hoped so, and then I said good-bye to Miss Scott in Spanish. The rough-looking attendant twisted his arms around mine, and half-led, half-dragged me to an ambulance. A crowd of the students had assembled, and they watched us curiously. I put the shawl over my face, and sank thankfully into the wagon. Miss Neville, Miss Mayard, Mrs. Fox, and Mrs. Schanz were all put in after me, one at a time. A man got in with us, the doors were locked, and we were driven out of the gates in great style on toward the Insane Asylum and victory! The patients made no move to escape. The odor of the male attendant's breath was enough to make one's head swim.

When we reached the wharf such a mob of people crowded around the wagon that the police were called to put them away, so that we could reach the boat. I was the last of the procession. I was escorted down the plank, the fresh breeze blowing the attendants' whisky breath into my face until I staggered. I was taken into a dirty cabin, where I found my companions seated on a narrow bench. The small windows were closed, and, with the smell of the filthy room, the air was stifling. At one end of the cabin was a small bunk in such a condition that I had to hold my nose when I went near it. A sick girl was put on it. An old woman, with an enormous bonnet and a dirty basket filled with chunks of bread and bits of scrap meat, completed our company. The door was guarded by two female attendants. One was clad in a dress made of bed-ticking and the other was dressed with some attempt at style. They were coarse, massive women, and expectorated tobacco juice about on the floor in a manner more skillful than charming. One of these fearful creatures seemed to have much faith in the power of the glance on insane people, for, when any one of us would move or go to look out of the high window she would say "Sit down," and would lower her brows and glare in a way that was simply terrifying.

While guarding the door they talked with some men on the outside. They discussed the number of patients and then their own affairs in a manner neither edifying nor refined.

ON BOARD THE ISLAND BOAT.

The boat stopped and the old woman and the sick girl were taken off. The rest of us were told to sit still. At the next stop my companions were taken off, one at a time. I was last, and it seemed to require a man and a woman to lead me up the plank to reach the shore. An ambulance was standing there, and in it were the four other patients.

"What is this place?" I asked of the man, who had his fingers sunk into the flesh of my arm.

"Blackwell's Island, an insane place, where you'll never get out of."

With this I was shoved into the ambulance, the springboard was put up, an officer and a mail-carrier jumped on behind, and I was swiftly driven to the Insane Asylum on Blackwell's Island.

CHAPTER VIII.
INSIDE THE MADHOUSE.

AS the wagon was rapidly driven through the beautiful lawns up to the asylum my feelings of satisfaction at having attained the object of my work were greatly dampened by the look of distress on the faces of my companions. Poor women, they had no hopes of a speedy delivery. They were being driven to a prison, through no fault of their own, in all probability for life. In comparison, how much easier it would be to walk to the gallows than to this tomb of living horrors! On the wagon sped, and I, as well as my comrades, gave a despairing farewell glance at freedom as we came in sight of the long stone buildings. We passed one low building, and the stench was so horrible that I was compelled to hold my breath, and I mentally decided that it was the kitchen. I afterward found I was correct in my surmise, and smiled at the signboard at the end of the walk: "Visitors are not allowed on this road." I don't think the sign would be necessary if they once tried the road, especially on a warm day.

The wagon stopped, and the nurse and officer in charge told us to get out. The nurse added: "Thank God! they came quietly." We obeyed orders to go ahead up a flight of narrow, stone steps, which had evidently been built for the accommodation of people who climb stairs three at a time. I wondered if my companions knew where we were, so I said to Miss Tillie Mayard:

"Where are we?"

"At the Blackwell's Island Lunatic Asylum," she answered, sadly.

"Are you crazy?" I asked.

"No," she replied; "but as we have been sent here we will have to be quiet until we find some means of escape. They will be few, though, if all the doctors, as Dr. Field, refuse to listen to me or give me a chance to prove my sanity." We were ushered into a narrow vestibule, and the door was locked behind us.

In spite of the knowledge of my sanity and the assurance that I would be released in a few days, my heart gave a sharp twinge. Pronounced insane by four expert doctors and shut up behind the unmerciful bolts and bars of a madhouse! Not to be confined alone, but to be a companion, day and night, of senseless, chattering lunatics; to sleep with them, to eat with them, to be considered one of them, was an uncomfortable position. Timidly we followed the nurse up the long uncarpeted hall to a room filled by so-called crazy women. We were told to sit down, and some of the patients kindly made room for us. They looked at us curiously, and one came up to me and asked:

"Who sent you here?"

"The doctors," I answered.

"What for?" she persisted.

"Well, they say I am insane," I admitted.

"Insane!" she repeated, incredulously. "It cannot be seen in your face."

This woman was too clever, I concluded, and was glad to answer the roughly given orders to follow the nurse to see the doctor. This nurse, Miss Grupe, by the way, had a nice German face, and if I had not detected certain hard lines about the mouth I might have expected, as did my companions, to receive but kindness from her. She left us in a small waiting-room at the end of the hall, and left us alone while she went into a small office opening into the sitting or receiving-room.

"I like to go down in the wagon," she said to the invisible party on the inside. "It helps to break up the day." He answered her that the open air improved her looks, and she again appeared before us all smiles and simpers.

THE INSANE ASYLUM.

"Come here, Tillie Mayard," she said. Miss Mayard obeyed, and, though I could not see into the office, I could hear her gently but firmly pleading her case. All her remarks were as rational as any I ever heard, and I thought no good physician could help but be impressed with her story. She told of her recent illness, that she was suffering from nervous debility. She begged that they try all their tests for insanity, if they had any, and give her justice. Poor girl, how my heart ached for her! I determined then and there that I would try by every means to make my mission of benefit to my suffering sisters; that I would show how they are committed without ample trial. Without one word of sympathy or encouragement she was brought back to where we sat.

Mrs. Louise Schanz was taken into the presence of Dr. Kinier, the medical man.

"Your name?" he asked, loudly. She answered in German, saying she did not speak English nor could she understand it. However, when he said Mrs. Louise Schanz, she said "Yah, yah." Then he tried other questions, and when he found she could not understand one world of English, he said to Miss Grupe:

"You are German; speak to her for me."

Miss Grupe proved to be one of those people who are ashamed of their nationality, and she refused, saying she could understand but few worlds of her mother tongue.

"You know you speak German. Ask this woman what her husband does," and they both laughed as if they were enjoying a joke.

44

"I can't speak but a few words," she protested, but at last she managed to ascertain the occupation of Mr. Schanz.

"Now, what was the use of lying to me?" asked the doctor, with a laugh which dispelled the rudeness.

"I can't speak any more," she said, and she did not.

Thus was Mrs. Louise Schanz consigned to the asylum without a chance of making herself understood. Can such carelessness be excused, I wonder, when it is so easy to get an interpreter? If the confinement was but for a few days one might question the necessity. But here was a woman taken without her own consent from the free world to an asylum and there given no chance to prove her sanity. Confined most probably for life behind asylum bars, without even being told in her language the why and wherefore. Compare this with a criminal, who is given every chance to prove his innocence. Who would not rather be a murderer and take the chance for life than be declared insane, without hope of escape? Mrs. Schanz begged in German to know where she was, and pleaded for liberty. Her voice broken by sobs, she was led unheard out to us.

THE FRONT HALLWAY.

Mrs. Fox was then put through this weak, trifling examination and brought from the office, convicted. Miss Annie Neville took her turn, and I was again left to the last. I had by this time determined to act as I do when free, except that I would refuse to tell who I was or where my home was.

CHAPTER IX.
AN EXPERT(?) AT WORK.

"NELLIE BROWN, the doctor wants you," said Miss Grupe. I went in and was told to sit down opposite Dr. Kinier at the desk.

"What is your name?" he asked, without looking up.

"Nellie Brown," I replied easily.

"Where is your home?" writing what I had said down in a large book.

"In Cuba."

"Oh!" he ejaculated, with sudden understanding–then, addressing the nurse:

"Did you see anything in the papers about her?"

"Yes," she replied, "I saw a long account of this girl in the *Sun* on Sunday." Then the doctor said:

"Keep her here until I go to the office and see the notice again."

He left us, and I was relieved of my hat and shawl. On his return, he said he had been unable to find the paper, but he related the story of my *debut*, as he had read it, to the nurse.

"What's the color of her eyes?"

Miss Grupe looked, and answered "gray," although everybody had always said my eyes were brown or hazel.

"What's your age?" he asked; and as I answered, "Nineteen last May," he turned to the nurse, and said, "When do you get your next pass?" This I ascertained was a leave of absence, or "a day off."

"Next Saturday," she said, with a laugh.

"You will go to town?" and they both laughed as she answered in the affirmative, and he said:

"Measure her." I was stood under a measure, and it was brought down tightly on my head.

"What is it?" asked the doctor.

"Now you know I can't tell," she said.

"Yes, you can; go ahead. What height?"

"I don't know; there are some figures there, but I can't tell."

"Yes, you can. Now look and tell me."

"I can't; do it yourself," and they laughed again as the doctor left his place at the desk and came forward to see for himself.

"Five feet five inches; don't you see?" he said, taking her hand and touching the figures.

By her voice I knew she did not understand yet, but that was no concern of mine, as the doctor seemed to find a pleasure in aiding her. Then I was put on the scales, and she worked around until she got them to balance.

"How much?" asked the doctor, having resumed his position at the desk.

"I don't know. You will have to see for yourself," she replied, calling him by his Christian name, which I have forgotten. He turned and also addressing her by her baptismal name, he said:

"You are getting too fresh!" and they both laughed. I then told the weight—112 pounds—to the nurse, and she in turn told the doctor.

"What time are you going to supper?" he asked, and she told him. He gave the nurse more attention than he did me, and asked her six questions to every one of me. Then he wrote my fate in the book before him. I said, "I am not sick and I do not want to stay here. No one has a right to shut me up in this manner." He took no notice of my remarks, and having completed his writings, as well as his talk with the nurse for the moment, he said that would do, and with my companions, I went back to the sitting-room.

"You play the piano?" they asked.

"Oh, yes; ever since I was a child," I replied.

Then they insisted that I should play, and they seated me on a wooden chair before an old-fashioned square. I struck a few notes, and the untuned response sent a grinding chill through me.

"How horrible," I exclaimed, turning to a nurse, Miss McCarten, who stood at my side. "I never touched a piano as much out of tune."

"It's a pity of you," she said, spitefully; "we'll have to get one made to order for you."

I began to play the variations of "Home Sweet Home." The talking ceased and every patient sat silent, while my cold fingers moved slowly and stiffly over the keyboard. I finished in an aimless fashion and refused all requests to play more. Not seeing an available place to sit, I still occupied the chair in the front of the piano while I "sized up" my surroundings.

It was a long, bare room, with bare yellow benches encircling it. These benches, which were perfectly straight, and just as uncomfortable, would hold five people, although in almost every instance six were crowded on them. Barred windows, built about five feet from the floor, faced the two double doors which led into the hall. The bare white walls were somewhat relieved by three lithographs, one of Fritz Emmet and the others of negro minstrels. In the center of the room was a large table covered with a white bed-spread, and around it sat the nurses. Everything was spotlessly clean and I thought what good workers the nurses must be to keep such order. In a few days after how I laughed at my own stupidity to think the nurses would work. When they found I would not play any more, Miss McCarten came up to me saying, roughly:

"Get away from here," and closed the piano with a bang.

"Brown, come here," was the next order I got from a rough, red-faced woman at the table. "What have you on?"

48

"My clothing," I replied.

She lifted my dress and skirts and wrote down one pair shoes, one pair stockings, one cloth dress, one straw sailor hat, and so on.

CHAPTER X.
MY FIRST SUPPER.

THIS examination over, we heard some one yell, "Go out into the hall." One of the patients kindly explained that this was an invitation to supper. We late comers tried to keep together, so we entered the hall and stood at the door where all the women had crowded. How we shivered as we stood there! The windows were open and the draught went whizzing through the hall. The patients looked blue with cold, and the minutes stretched into a quarter of an hour. At last one of the nurses went forward and unlocked a door, through which we all crowded to a landing of the stairway. Here again came a long halt directly before an open window.

"How very imprudent for the attendants to keep these thinly clad women standing here in the cold," said Miss Neville.

I looked at the poor crazy captives shivering, and added, emphatically, "It's horribly brutal." While they stood there I thought I would not relish supper that night. They looked so lost and hopeless. Some were chattering nonsense to invisible persons, others were laughing or crying aimlessly, and one old, gray-haired woman was nudging me, and, with winks and sage noddings of the head and pitiful uplifting of the eyes and hands, was assuring me that I must not mind the poor creatures, as they were all mad. "Stop at the heater," was then ordered, "and get in line, two by two." "Mary, get a companion." "How many times must I tell you to keep in line?" "Stand still," and, as the orders were issued, a shove and a push were administered, and often a slap on the ears. After this third and final halt, we were marched into a long, narrow dining-room, where a rush was made for the table.

The table reached the length of the room and was uncovered and uninviting. Long benches without backs were put for the patients to sit on, and over these they had to crawl in order to face the table. Placed closed together all along the table were large dressing-bowls filled with a pinkish-looking stuff which the patients called tea. By each bowl was laid a piece of bread, cut thick and buttered. A small saucer containing five prunes accompanied the bread. One fat woman made a rush, and jerking up several saucers from those around her emptied their contents into her own saucer. Then while holding to her own bowl she lifted up another and drained its contents at one gulp. This she did to a second bowl in shorter time than it takes to tell it. Indeed, I was so amused at her successful grabbings that when I looked at my own share the woman opposite, without so much as by your leave, grabbed my bread and left me without any.

Another patient, seeing this, kindly offered me hers, but I declined with thanks and turned to the nurse and asked for more. As she flung a thick piece down on the table she made some remark about the fact that if I forgot where my home was I had not forgotten how to eat. I tried the bread, but the butter was so horrible that one could not eat it. A blue-eyed German girl on the opposite side of the table told me I could have bread unbuttered if I wished, and that very few were able to eat the butter. I turned my attention to the prunes and found that very few of them would be sufficient. A patient near asked me to give them to her. I did so. My bowl of tea was all that was left. I tasted, and one taste was enough. It had no sugar, and it tasted as if it had been made in copper. It was as weak as water. This was also transferred to a hungrier patient, in spite of the protest of Miss Neville.

"You must force the food down," she said, "else you will be sick, and who know but what, with these surroundings, you may go crazy. To have a good brain the stomach must be cared for."

"It is impossible for me to eat that stuff," I replied, and, despite all her urging, I ate nothing that night.

It did not require much time for the patients to consume all that was eatable on the table, and then we got our orders to form in line in the hall. When this was done the doors before us were unlocked and we were ordered to proceed back to the sitting-room. Many of the patients crowded near us, and I was again urged to play, both by them and by the nurses. To please the patients I promised to play and Miss Tillie Mayard was to sing. The first thing she asked me to play was "Rock-a-bye Baby," and I did so. She sang it beautifully.

CHAPTER XI.
IN THE BATH.

A FEW more songs and we were told to go with Miss Grupe. We were taken into a cold, wet bathroom, and I was ordered to undress. Did I protest? Well, I never grew so earnest in my life as when I tried to beg off. They said if I did not they would use force and that it would not be very gentle. At this I noticed one of the craziest women in the ward standing by the filled bathtub with a large, discolored rag in her hands. She was chattering away to herself and chuckling in a manner which seemed to me fiendish. I knew now what was to be done with me. I shivered. They began to undress me, and one by one they pulled off my clothes. At last everything was gone excepting one garment. "I will not remove it," I said vehemently, but they took it off. I gave one glance at the group of patients gathered at the door watching the scene, and I jumped into the bathtub with more energy than grace.

THE RECEPTION-ROOM.

The water was ice-cold, and I again began to protest. How useless it all was! I begged, at least, that the patients be made to go away, but was ordered to shut up. The crazy woman began to scrub me. I can find no other word that will express it but scrubbing. From a small tin pan she took some soft soap and rubbed it all over me, even all over my face and my pretty hair. I was at last past seeing or speaking, although I had begged that my hair be left untouched. Rub, rub, rub, went the old woman, chattering to herself. My teeth chattered and my limbs were goose-fleshed and blue with cold. Suddenly I got, one after the other, three buckets of water over my head–ice-cold water, too–into my eyes, my ears, my nose and my mouth. I think I experienced some of the sensations of a drowning person as they dragged me, gasping, shivering and quaking, from the tub.

52

For once I did look insane. I caught a glance of the indescribable look on the faces of my companions, who had witnessed my fate and knew theirs was surely following. Unable to control myself at the absurd picture I presented, I burst into roars of laughter. They put me, dripping wet, into a short canton flannel slip, labeled across the extreme end in large black letters, "Lunatic Asylum, B. I., H. 6." The letters meant Blackwell's Island, Hall 6.

By this time Miss Mayard had been undressed, and, much as I hated my recent bath, I would have taken another if by it I could have saved her the experience. Imagine plunging that sick girl into a cold bath when it made me, who have never been ill, shake as if with ague. I heard her explain to Miss Grupe that her head was still sore from her illness. Her hair was short and had mostly come out, and she asked that the crazy woman be made to rub more gently, but Miss Grupe said:

"There isn't much fear of hurting you. Shut up, or you'll get it worse." Miss Mayard did shut up, and that was my last look at her for the night.

I was hurried into a room where there were six beds, and had been put into bed when some one came along and jerked me out again, saying:

"Nellie Brown has to be put in a room alone to-night, for I suppose she's noisy."

I was taken to room 28 and left to try and make an impression on the bed. It was an impossible task. The bed had been made high in the center and sloping on either side. At the first touch my head flooded the pillow with water, and my wet slip transferred some of its dampness to the sheet. When Miss Grupe came in I asked if I could not have a night-gown.

"We have not such things in this institution," she said.

"I do not like to sleep without," I replied.

"Well, I don't care about that," she said. "You are in a public institution now, and you can't expect to get anything. This is charity, and you should be thankful for what you get."

"But the city pays to keep these places up," I urged, "and pays people to be kind to the unfortunates brought here."

"Well, you don't need to expect any kindness here, for you won't get it," she said, and she went out and closed the door.

HER BEDROOM.

A sheet and an oilcloth were under me, and a sheet and black wool blanket above. I never felt anything so annoying as that wool blanket as I tried to keep it around my shoulders to stop the chills from getting underneath. When I pulled it up I left my feet bare, and when I pulled it down my shoulders were exposed. There was absolutely nothing in the room but the bed and myself. As the door had been locked I imagined I should be left alone for the night, but I heard the sound of the heavy tread of two women down the hall. They stopped at every door, unlocked it, and in a few moments I could hear them relock it. This they did without the least attempt at quietness down the whole length of the opposite side of the hall and up to my room. Here they paused. The key was inserted in the lock and turned. I watched those about to enter. In they came, dressed in brown and white striped dresses, fastened by brass buttons, large, white aprons, a heavy green cord about the waist, from which dangled a bunch of large keys, and small, white caps on their heads. Being dressed as were the attendants of the day, I knew they were nurses. The first one carried a lantern, and she flashed its light into my face while she said to her assistant:

"This is Nellie Brown." Looking at her, I asked:

"Who are you?"

"The night nurse, my dear," she replied, and, wishing that I would sleep well, she went out and locked the door after her. Several times during the night they came into my room, and even had I been able to sleep, the unlocking of the heavy door, their loud talking, and heavy tread, would have awakened me.

I could not sleep, so I lay in bed picturing to myself the horrors in case a fire should break out in the asylum. Every door is locked separately and the windows are heavily barred, so that escape is impossible. In the one building alone there are, I think Dr. Ingram told me, some three hundred women. They are locked, one to ten to a room. It is impossible to get out unless these doors are unlocked. A fire is not improbable, but one of the most likely occurrences. Should the building burn, the jailers or nurses would never think of releasing their crazy patients. This I can prove to you later when I come to tell of their cruel treatment of the poor things intrusted to their care. As I say, in case of fire, not a dozen women could escape. All would be left to roast to death. Even if the nurses were kind, which they are not, it would require more presence of mind than women of their class possess to risk the flames and their own lives while they unlocked the hundred doors for the insane prisoners. Unless there is a change there will some day be a tale of horror never equaled.

In this connection is an amusing incident which happened just previous to my release. I was talking with Dr. Ingram about many things, and at last told him what I thought would be the result of a fire.

"The nurses are expected to open the doors," he said.

"But you know positively that they would not wait to do that," I said, "and these women would burn to death."

He sat silent, unable to contradict my assertion.

"Why don't you have it changed?" I asked.

"What can I do?" he replied. "I offer suggestions until my brain is tired, but what good does it do? What would you do?" he asked, turning to me, the proclaimed insane girl.

"Well, I should insist on them having locks put in, as I have seen in some places, that by turning a crank at the end of the hall you can lock or unlock

55

every door on the one side. Then there would be some chance of escape. Now, every door being locked separately, there is absolutely none."

Dr. Ingram turned to me with an anxious look on his kind face as he asked, slowly:

"Nellie Brown, what institution have you been an inmate of before you came here?"

"None. I never was confined in any institution, except boarding-school, in my life."

"Where then did you see the locks you have described?"

I had seen them in the new Western Penitentiary at Pittsburg, Pa., but I did not dare say so. I merely answered:

"Oh, I have seen them in a place I was in–I mean as a visitor."

"There is only one place I know of where they have those locks," he said, sadly, "and that is at Sing Sing."

The inference is conclusive. I laughed very heartily over the implied accusation, and tried to assure him that I had never, up to date, been an inmate of Sing Sing or even ever visited it.

Just as the morning began to dawn I went to sleep. It did not seem many moments until I was rudely awakened and told to get up, the window being opened and the clothing pulled off me. My hair was still wet and I had pains all through me, as if I had the rheumatism. Some clothing was flung on the floor and I was told to put it on. I asked for my own, but was told to take what I got and keep quiet by the apparently head nurse, Miss Grady. I looked at it. One underskirt made of coarse dark cotton goods and a cheap white calico dress with a black spot in it. I tied the strings of the skirt around me and put on the little dress. It was made, as are all those worn by the patients, into a straight tight waist sewed on to a straight skirt. As I buttoned the waist I noticed the underskirt was about six inches longer than the upper, and for a moment I sat down on the bed and laughed at my own appearance. No woman ever longed for a mirror more than I did at that moment.

I saw the other patients hurrying past in the hall, so I decided not to lose anything that might be going on. We numbered forty-five patients in Hall 6, and were sent to the bathroom, where there were two coarse towels. I watched crazy patients who had the most dangerous eruptions all over their faces dry on the towels and then saw women with clean skins turn to use them. I went to the bathtub and washed my face at the running faucet and my underskirt did duty for a towel.

Before I had completed my ablutions a bench was brought into the bathroom. Miss Grupe and Miss McCarten came in with combs in their hands. We were told so sit down on the bench, and the hair of forty-five women was combed with one patient, two nurses, and six combs. As I saw some of the sore heads combed I thought this was another dose I had not bargained for. Miss Tillie Mayard had her own comb, but it was taken from her by Miss Grady. Oh, that combing! I never realized before what the expression "I'll give you a combing" meant, but I knew then. My hair, all matted and wet from the night previous, was pulled and jerked, and, after expostulating to no avail, I set my teeth and endured the pain. They refused to give me my hairpins, and my hair was arranged in one plait and tied with a red cotton rag. My curly bangs refused to stay back, so that at least was left of my former glory.

After this we went to the sitting-room and I looked for my companions. At first I looked vainly, unable to distinguish them from the other patients, but after awhile I recognized Miss Mayard by her short hair.

"How did you sleep after your cold bath?"

"I almost froze, and then the noise kept me awake. It's dreadful! My nerves were so unstrung before I came here, and I fear I shall not be able to stand the strain."

I did the best I could to cheer her. I asked that we be given additional clothing, at least as much as custom says women shall wear, but they told me to shut up; that we had as much as they intended to give us.

We were compelled to get up at 5.30 o'clock, and at 7.15 we were told to collect in the hall, where the experience of waiting, as on the evening previous, was repeated. When we got into the dining-room at last we found a bowl of cold tea, a slice of buttered bread and a saucer of oatmeal, with molasses on it, for each patient. I was hungry, but the food would not down. I asked for unbuttered bread and was given it. I cannot tell you of anything which is the same dirty, black color. It was hard, and in places nothing more than dried dough. I found a spider in my slice, so I did not eat it. I tried the oatmeal and molasses, but it was wretched, and so I endeavored, but without much show of success, to choke down the tea.

After we were back to the sitting-room a number of women were ordered to make the beds, and some of the patients were put to scrubbing and others given different duties which covered all the work in the hall. It is not the attendants who keep the institution so nice for the poor patients, as I had always thought, but the patients, who do it all themselves–even to cleaning the nurses' bedrooms and caring for their clothing.

About 9.30 the new patients, of which I was one, were told to go out to see the doctor. I was taken in and my lungs and my heart were examined by the flirty young doctor who was the first to see us the day we entered. The one who made out the report, if I mistake not, was the assistant superintendent, Ingram. A few questions and I was allowed to return to the sitting-room.

I came in and saw Miss Grady with my note-book and long lead pencil, bought just for the occasion.

"I want my book and pencil," I said, quite truthfully. "It helps me remember things."

I was very anxious to get it to make notes in and was disappointed when she said:

"You can't have it, so shut up."

Some days after I asked Dr. Ingram if I could have it, and he promised to consider the matter. When I again referred to it, he said that Miss Grady said I only brought a book there; and that I had no pencil. I was provoked, and insisted that I had, whereupon I was advised to fight against the imaginations of my brain.

After the housework was completed by the patients, and as day was fine, but cold, we were told to go out in the hall and get on shawls and hats for a walk. Poor patients! How eager they were for a breath of air; how eager for a slight release from their prison. They went swiftly into the hall and there was a skirmish for hats. Such hats!

AN INSANE HALL.

CHAPTER XII.
PROMENADING WITH LUNATICS.

I SHALL never forget my first walk. When all the patients had donned the white straw hats, such as bathers wear at Coney Island, I could not but laugh at their comical appearances. I could not distinguish one woman from another. I lost Miss Neville, and had to take my hat off and search for her. When we met we put our hats on and laughed at one another. Two by two we formed in line, and guarded by the attendants we went out a back way on to the walks.

We had not gone many paces when I saw, proceeding from every walk, long lines of women guarded by nurses. How many there were! Every way I looked I could see them in the queer dresses, comical straw hats and shawls, marching slowly around. I eagerly watched the passing lines and a thrill of horror crept over me at the sight. Vacant eyes and meaningless faces, and their tongues uttered meaningless nonsense. One crowd passed and I noted by nose as well as eyes, that they were fearfully dirty.

"Who are they?" I asked of a patient near me.

"They are considered the most violent on the island," she replied. "They are from the Lodge, the first building with the high steps." Some were yelling, some were cursing, others were singing or praying or preaching, as the fancy struck them, and they made up the most miserable collection of humanity I had ever seen. As the din of their passing faded in the distance there came another sight I can never forget:

A long cable rope fastened to wide leather belts, and these belts locked around the waists of fifty-two women. At the end of the rope was a heavy iron cart, and in it two women—one nursing a sore foot, another screaming at some nurse, saying: "You beat me and I shall not forget it. You want to kill me," and then she would sob and cry. The women "on the rope," as the patients call it, were each busy on their individual freaks. Some were yelling all the while. One who had blue eyes saw me look at her, and she turned as far as she could, talking and smiling, with that terrible, horrifying look of absolute insanity stamped on her. The doctors might safely judge on her case. The horror of that sight to one who had never been near an insane person before, was something unspeakable.

"God help them!" breathed Miss Neville. "It is so dreadful I cannot look."

On they passed, but for their places to be filled by more. Can you imagine the sight? According to one of the physicians there are 1600 insane women on Blackwell's Island.

Mad! what can be half so horrible? My heart thrilled with pity when I looked on old, gray-haired women talking aimlessly to space. One woman had on a straightjacket, and two women had to drag her along. Crippled, blind, old, young, homely, and pretty; one senseless mass of humanity. No fate could be worse.

I looked at the pretty lawns, which I had once thought was such a comfort to the poor creatures confined on the Island, and laughed at my own notions. What enjoyment is it to them? They are not allowed on the grass— it is only to look at. I saw some patients eagerly and caressingly lift a nut or a colored leaf that had fallen on the path. But they were not permitted to keep them. The nurses would always compel them to throw their little bit of God's comfort away.

QUIET INMATES OUT FOR A WALK. As I passed a low pavilion, where a crowd of helpless lunatics were confined, I read a motto on the wall, "While I live I hope." The absurdity of it struck me forcibly. I would have liked to put above the gates that open to the asylum, "He who enters here leaveth hope behind."

61

During the walk I was annoyed a great deal by nurses who had heard my romantic story calling to those in charge of us to ask which one I was. I was pointed out repeatedly.

It was not long until the dinner hour arrived and I was so hungry that I felt I could eat anything. The same old story of standing for a half and three-quarters of an hour in the hall was repeated before we got down to our dinners. The bowls in which we had had our tea were now filled with soup, and on a plate was one cold boiled potato and a chunk of beef, which on investigation, proved to be slightly spoiled. There were no knives or forks, and the patients looked fairly savage as they took the tough beef in their fingers and pulled in opposition to their teeth. Those toothless or with poor teeth could not eat it. One tablespoon was given for the soup, and a piece of bread was the final entree. Butter is never allowed at dinner nor coffee or tea. Miss Mayard could not eat, and I saw many of the sick ones turn away in disgust. I was getting very weak from the want of food and tried to eat a slice of bread. After the first few bites hunger asserted itself, and I was able to eat all but the crusts of the one slice.

Superintendent Dent went through the sitting-room, giving an occasional "How do you do?" "How are you to-day?" here and there among the patients. His voice was as cold as the hall, and the patients made no movement to tell him of their sufferings. I asked some of them to tell how they were suffering from the cold and insufficiency of clothing, but they replied that the nurse would beat them if they told.

I was never so tired as I grew sitting on those benches. Several of the patients would sit on one foot or sideways to make a change, but they were always reproved and told to sit up straight. If they talked they were scolded and told to shut up; if they wanted to walk around in order to take the stiffness out of them, they were told to sit down and be still. What, excepting torture, would produce insanity quicker than this treatment? Here is a class of women sent to be cured. I would like the expert physicians who are condemning me for my action, which has proven their ability, to take a perfectly sane and healthy woman, shut her up and make her sit from 6 A. M. until 8 P. M. on straight-back benches, do not allow her to talk or move during these hours, give her no reading and let her know nothing of the world or its doings, give her bad food and harsh treatment, and see how long it will take to make her insane. Two months would make her a mental and physical wreck.

I have described my first day in the asylum, and as my other nine were exactly the same in the general run of things it would be tiresome to tell about each. In giving this story I expect to be contradicted by many who are exposed. I merely tell in common words, without exaggeration, of my life in a mad-house for ten days. The eating was one of the most horrible things. Excepting the first two days after I entered the asylum, there was no salt for the food. The hungry and even famishing women made an attempt to eat the horrible messes. Mustard and vinegar were put on meat and in soup to give it a taste, but it only helped to make it worse. Even that was all consumed after two days, and the patients had to try to choke down fresh fish, just boiled in water, without salt, pepper or butter; mutton, beef and potatoes without the faintest seasoning. The most insane refused to swallow the food and were threatened with punishment. In our short walks we passed the kitchen were food was prepared for the nurses and doctors. There we got glimpses of melons and grapes and all kinds of fruits, beautiful white bread and nice meats, and the hungry feeling would be increased tenfold. I spoke to some of the physicians, but it had no effect, and when I was taken away the food was yet unsalted.

My heart ached to see the sick patients grow sicker over the table. I saw Miss Tillie Mayard so suddenly overcome at a bite that she had to rush from the dining-room and then got a scolding for doing so. When the patients complained of the food they were told to shut up; that they would not have as good if they were at home, and that it was too good for charity patients.

A German girl, Louise–I have forgotten her last name–did not eat for several days and at last one morning she was missing. From the conversation of the nurses I found she was suffering from a high fever. Poor thing! she told me she unceasingly prayed for death. I watched the nurses make a patient carry such food as the well ones were refusing up to Louise's room. Think of that stuff for a fever patient! Of course, she refused it. Then I saw a nurse, Miss McCarten, go to test her temperature, and she returned with a report of it being some 150 degrees. I smiled at the report, and Miss Grupe, seeing it, asked me how high my temperature had ever run. I refused to answer. Miss Grady then decided to try her ability. She returned with the report of 99 degrees.

Miss Tillie Mayard suffered more than any of us from the cold, and yet she tried to follow my advice to be cheerful and try to keep up for a short time. Superintendent Dent brought in a man to see me. He felt my pulse and my head and examined my tongue. I told them how cold it was, and assured them that I did not need medical aid, but that Miss Mayard did, and they should transfer their attentions to her. They did not answer me, and I was pleased to see Miss Mayard leave her place and come forward to them. She spoke to the doctors and told them she was ill, but they paid no attention to her. The nurses came and dragged her back to the bench, and after the doctors left they said, "After awhile, when you see that the doctors will not notice you, you will quit running up to them." Before the doctors left me I heard one say–I cannot give it in his exact words–that my pulse and eyes were not that of an insane girl, but Superintendent Dent assured him that in cases such as mine such tests failed. After watching me for awhile he said my face was the brightest he had ever seen for a lunatic. The nurses had on heavy undergarments and coats, but they refused to give us shawls.

Nearly all night long I listened to a woman cry about the cold and beg for God to let her die. Another one yelled "Murder!" at frequent intervals and "Police!" at others until my flesh felt creepy.

The second morning, after we had begun our endless "set" for the day, two of the nurses, assisted by some patients, brought the woman in who had begged the night previous for God to take her home. I was not surprised at her prayer. She appeared easily seventy years old, and she was blind. Although the halls were freezing-cold, that old woman had no more clothing on than the rest of us, which I have described. When she was brought into the sitting-room and placed on the hard bench, she cried:

"Oh, what are you doing with me? I am cold, so cold. Why can't I stay in bed or have a shawl?" and then she would get up and endeavor to feel her way to leave the room. Sometimes the attendants would jerk her back to the bench, and again they would let her walk and heartlessly laugh when she bumped against the table or the edge of the benches. At one time she said the heavy shoes which charity provides hurt her feet, and she took them off. The nurses made two patients put them on her again, and when she did it several times, and fought against having them on, I counted seven people at her at once trying to put the shoes on her. The old woman then tried to lie down on the bench, but they pulled her up again. It sounded so pitiful to hear her cry:

"Oh, give me a pillow and pull the covers over me, I am so cold."

At this I saw Miss Grupe sit down on her and run her cold hands over the old woman's face and down inside the neck of her dress. At the old woman's cries she laughed savagely, as did the other nurses, and repeated her cruel action. That day the old woman was carried away to another ward.

CHAPTER XIII.
CHOKING AND BEATING PATIENTS.

MISS TILLIE MAYARD suffered greatly from cold. One morning she sat on the bench next to me and was livid with the cold. Her limbs shook and her teeth chattered. I spoke to the three attendants who sat with coats on at the table in the center of the floor.

"It is cruel to lock people up and then freeze them," I said. They replied she had on as much as any of the rest, and she would get no more. Just then Miss Mayard took a fit and every patient looked frightened. Miss Neville caught her in her arms and held her, although the nurses roughly said:

"Let her fall on the floor and it will teach her a lesson." Miss Neville told them what she thought of their actions, and then I got orders to make my appearance in the office.

Just as I reached there Superintendent Dent came to the door and I told him how we were suffering from the cold, and of Miss Mayard's condition. Doubtless, I spoke incoherently, for I told of the state of the food, the treatment of the nurses and their refusal to give more clothing, the condition of Miss Mayard, and the nurses telling us, because the asylum was a public institution we could not expect even kindness. Assuring him that I needed no medical aid, I told him to go to Miss Mayard. He did so. From Miss Neville and other patients I learned what transpired. Miss Mayard was still in the fit, and he caught her roughly between the eyebrows or thereabouts, and pinched until her face was crimson from the rush of blood to the head, and her senses returned. All day afterward she suffered from terrible headache, and from that on she grew worse.

Insane? Yes, insane; and as I watched the insanity slowly creep over the mind that had appeared to be all right I secretly cursed the doctors, the nurses and all public institutions. Some one may say that she was insane at some time previous to her consignment to the asylum. Then if she were, was this the proper place to send a woman just convalescing, to be given cold baths, deprived of sufficient clothing and fed with horrible food?

On this morning I had a long conversation with Dr. Ingram, the assistant superintendent of the asylum. I found that he was kind to the helpless in

66

his charge. I began my old complaint of the cold, and he called Miss Grady to the office and ordered more clothing given the patients. Miss Grady said if I made a practice of telling it would be a serious thing for me, she warned me in time.

Many visitors looking for missing girls came to see me. Miss Grady yelled in the door from the hall one day:

"Nellie Brown, you're wanted."

I went to the sitting-room at the end of the hall, and there sat a gentleman who had known me intimately for years. I saw by the sudden blanching of his face and his inability to speak that the sight of me was wholly unexpected and had shocked him terribly. In an instant I determined, if he betrayed me as Nellie Bly, to say I had never seen him before. However, I had one card to play and I risked it. With Miss Grady within touching distance I whispered hurriedly to him, in language more expressive than elegant:

"Don't give me away."

I knew by the expression of his eye that he understood, so I said to Miss Grady:

"I do not know this man."

"Do you know her?" asked Miss Grady.

"No; this is not the young lady I came in search of," he replied, in a strained voice.

"If you do not know her you cannot stay here," she said, and she took him to the door. All at once a fear struck me that he would think I had been sent there through some mistake and would tell my friends and make an effort to have me released. So I waited until Miss Grady had the door unlocked. I knew that she would have to lock it before she could leave, and the time required to do so would give me opportunity to speak, so I called:

"One moment, senor." He returned to me and I asked aloud:

"Do you speak Spanish, senor?" and then whispered, "It's all right. I'm after an item. Keep still." "No," he said, with a peculiar emphasis, which I knew meant that he would keep my secret.

People in the world can never imagine the length of days to those in asylums. They seemed never ending, and we welcomed any event that might give us something to think about as well as talk of. There is nothing to read, and the only bit of talk that never wears out is conjuring up delicate food that they will get as soon as they get out. Anxiously the hour was watched for when the boat arrived to see if there were any new unfortunates to be added to our ranks. When they came and were ushered into the sitting-room the patients would express sympathy to one another for them and were anxious to show them little marks of attention. Hall 6 was the receiving hall, so that was how we saw all newcomers.

Soon after my advent a girl called Urena Little-Page was brought in. She was, as she had been born, silly, and her tender spot was, as with many sensible women, her age. She claimed eighteen, and would grow very angry if told to the contrary. The nurses were not long in finding this out, and then they teased her.

"Urena," said Miss Grady, "the doctors say that you are thirty-three instead of eighteen," and the other nurses laughed. They kept up this until the simple creature began to yell and cry, saying she wanted to go home and that everybody treated her badly. After they had gotten all the amusement out of her they wanted and she was crying, they began to scold and tell her to keep quiet. She grew more hysterical every moment until they pounced upon her and slapped her face and knocked her head in a lively fashion. This made the poor creature cry the more, and so they choked her. Yes, actually choked her. Then they dragged her out to the closet, and I heard her terrified cries hush into smothered ones. After several hours' absence she returned to the sitting-room, and I plainly saw the marks of their fingers on her throat for the entire day.

This punishment seemed to awaken their desire to administer more. They returned to the sitting-room and caught hold of an old gray-haired woman whom I have heard addressed both as Mrs. Grady and Mrs. O'Keefe. She was insane, and she talked almost continually to herself and to those near her. She never spoke very loud, and at the time I speak of was sitting harmlessly chattering to herself. They grabbed her, and my heart ached as she cried:

"For God sake, ladies, don't let them beat me."

"Shut up, you hussy!" said Miss Grady as she caught the woman by her gray hair and dragged her shrieking and pleading from the room. She was also taken to the closet, and her cries grew lower and lower, and then ceased.

The nurses returned to the room and Miss Grady remarked that she had "settled the old fool for awhile." I told some of the physicians of the occurrence, but they did not pay any attention to it.

One of the characters in Hall 6 was Matilda, a little old German woman, who, I believe, went insane over the loss of money. She was small, and had a pretty pink complexion. She was not much trouble, except at times. She would take spells, when she would talk into the steam-heaters or get up on a chair and talk out of the windows. In these conversations she railed at the lawyers who had taken her property. The nurses seemed to find a great deal of amusement in teasing the harmless old soul. One day I sat beside Miss Grady and Miss Grupe, and heard them tell her perfectly vile things to call Miss McCarten. After telling her to say these things they would send her to the other nurse, but Matilda proved that she, even in her state, had more sense than they.

"I cannot tell you. It is private," was all she would say. I saw Miss Grady, on a pretense of whispering to her, spit in her ear. Matilda quietly wiped her ear and said nothing.

CHAPTER XIV.
SOME UNFORTUNATE STORIES.

BY this time I had made the acquaintance of the greater number of the forty-five women in hall 6. Let me introduce a few. Louise, the pretty German girl who I have spoken of formerly as being sick with fever, had the delusion that the spirits of her dead parents were with her. "I have gotten many beatings from Miss Grady and her assistants," she said, "and I am unable to eat the horrible food they give us. I ought not to be compelled to freeze for want of proper clothing. Oh! I pray nightly that I may be taken to my papa and mamma. One night, when I was confined at Bellevue, Dr. Field came; I was in bed, and weary of the examination. At last I said: 'I am tired of this. I will talk no more.' 'Won't you?' he said, angrily. 'I'll see if I can't make you.' With this he laid his crutch on the side of the bed, and, getting up on it, he pinched me very severely in the ribs. I jumped up straight in bed, and said: 'What do you mean by this?' 'I want to teach you to obey when I speak to you,' he replied. If I could only die and go to papa!" When I left she was confined to bed with a fever, and maybe by this time she has her wish.

There is a Frenchwoman confined in hall 6, or was during my stay, whom I firmly believe to be perfectly sane. I watched her and talked with her every day, excepting the last three, and I was unable to find any delusion or mania in her. Her name is Josephine Despreau, if that is spelled correctly, and her husband and all her friends are in France. Josephine feels her position keenly. Her lips tremble, and she breaks down crying when she talks of her helpless condition. "How did you get here?" I asked.

"One morning as I was trying to get breakfast I grew deathly sick, and two officers were called in by the woman of the house, and I was taken to the station-house. I was unable to understand their proceedings, and they paid little attention to my story. Doings in this country were new to me, and before I realized it I was lodged as an insane woman in this asylum. When I first came I cried that I was here without hope of release, and for crying Miss Grady and her assistants choked me until they hurt my throat, for it has been sore ever since."

A pretty young Hebrew woman spoke so little English I could not get her story except as told by the nurses. They said her name is Sarah Fishbaum, and that her husband put her in the asylum because she had a fondness for other men than himself. Granting that Sarah was insane, and about men, let me tell you how the nurses tried to cure(?) her. They would call her up and say:

"Sarah, wouldn't you like to have a nice young man?"

"Oh, yes; a young man is all right," Sarah would reply in her few English words.

"Well, Sarah, wouldn't you like us to speak a good word to some of the doctors for you? Wouldn't you like to have one of the doctors?"

And then they would ask her which doctor she preferred, and advise her to make advances to him when he visited the hall, and so on.

I had been watching and talking with a fair-complexioned woman for several days, and I was at a loss to see why she had been sent there, she was so sane.

"Why did you come here?" I asked her one day, after we had indulged in a long conversation.

"I was sick," she replied.

"Are you sick mentally?" I urged.

"Oh, no; what gave you such an idea? I had been overworking myself, and I broke down. Having some family trouble, and being penniless and nowhere to go, I applied to the commissioners to be sent to the poorhouse until I would be able to go to work."

"But they do not send poor people here unless they are insane," I said. "Don't you know there are only insane women, or those supposed to be so, sent here?"

"I knew after I got here that the majority of these women were insane, but then I believed them when they told me this was the place they sent all the poor who applied for aid as I had done."

"How have you been treated?" I asked. "Well, so far I have escaped a beating, although I have been sickened at the sight of many and the recital of more. When I was brought here they went to give me a bath, and the very disease for which I needed doctoring and from which I was suffering made it necessary that I should not bathe. But they put me in, and my sufferings were increased greatly for weeks thereafter."

A Mrs. McCartney, whose husband is a tailor, seems perfectly rational and has not one fancy. Mary Hughes and Mrs. Louise Schanz showed no obvious traces of insanity.

One day two new-comers were added to our list. The one was an idiot, Carrie Glass, and the other was a nice-looking German girl–quite young, she seemed, and when she came in all the patients spoke of her nice appearance and apparent sanity. Her name was Margaret. She told me she had been a cook, and was extremely neat. One day, after she had scrubbed the kitchen floor, the chambermaids came down and deliberately soiled it. Her temper was aroused and she began to quarrel with them; an officer was called and she was taken to an asylum.

"How can they say I am insane, merely because I allowed my temper to run away with me?" she complained. "Other people are not shut up for crazy when they get angry. I suppose the only thing to do is to keep quiet and so avoid the beatings which I see others get. No one can say one word about me. I do everything I am told, and all the work they give me. I am obedient in every respect, and I do everything to prove to them that I am sane."

One day an insane woman was brought in. She was noisy, and Miss Grady gave her a beating and blacked her eye. When the doctors noticed it and asked if it was done before she came there the nurses said it was.

While I was in hall 6 I never heard the nurses address the patients except to scold or yell at them, unless it was to tease the. They spent much of their time gossiping about the physicians and about the other nurses in a manner that was not elevating. Miss Grady nearly always interspersed her conversation with profane language, and generally began her sentences by calling on the name of the Lord. The names she called the patients were of the lowest and most profane type. One evening she quarreled with another nurse while we were at supper about the bread, and when the nurse had gone out she called her bad names and made ugly remarks about her.

In the evenings a woman, whom I supposed to be head cook for the doctors, used to come up and bring raisins, grapes, apples, and crackers to the nurses. Imagine the feelings of the hungry patients as they sat and watched the nurses eat what was to them a dream of luxury.

One afternoon, Dr. Dent was talking to a patient, Mrs. Turney, about some trouble she had had with a nurse or matron. A short time after we were taken down to supper and this woman who had beaten Mrs. Turney, and of whom Dr. Dent spoke, was sitting at the door of our dining-room. Suddenly Mrs. Turney picked up her bowl of tea, and, rushing out of the door flung it at the woman who had beat her. There was some loud screaming and Mrs. Turney was returned to her place. The next day she was transferred to the "rope gang," which is supposed to be composed of the most dangerous and most suicidal women on the island.

At first I could not sleep and did not want to so long as I could hear anything new. The night nurses may have complained of the fact. At any rate one night they came in and tried to make me take a dose of some mixture out of a glass "to make me sleep," they said. I told them I would do nothing of the sort and they left me, I hoped, for the night. My hopes were vain, for in a few minutes they returned with a doctor, the same that received us on our arrival. He insisted that I take it, but I was determined not to lose my wits even for a few hours. When he saw that I was not to be coaxed he grew rather rough, and said he had wasted too much time with me already. That if I did not take it he would put it into my arm with a needle. It occurred to me that if he put it into my arm I could not get rid of it, but if I swallowed it there was one hope, so I said I would take it. I smelt it and it smelt like laudanum, and it was a horrible dose. No sooner had they left the room and locked me in than I tried so see how far down my throat my finger would go, and the chloral was allowed to try its effect elsewhere.

I want to say that the night nurse, Burns, in hall 6, seemed very kind and patient to the poor, afflicted people. The other nurses made several attempts to talk to me about lovers, and asked me if I would not like to have one. They did not find me very communicative on the–to them– popular subject.

Once a week the patients are given a bath, and that is the only time they see soap. A patient handed me a piece of soap one day about the size of a thimble, I considered it a great compliment in her wanting to be kind, but

I thought she would appreciate the cheap soap more than I, so I thanked her but refused to take it. On bathing day the tub is filled with water, and the patients are washed, one after the other, without a change of water. This is done until the water is really thick, and then it is allowed to run out and the tub is refilled without being washed. The same towels are used on all the women, those with eruptions as well as those without. The healthy patients fight for a change of water, but they are compelled to submit to the dictates of the lazy, tyrannical nurses. The dresses are seldom changed oftener than once a month. If the patient has a visitor, I have seen the nurses hurry her out and change her dress before the visitor comes in. This keeps up the appearance of careful and good management.

The patients who are not able to take care of themselves get into beastly conditions, and the nurses never look after them, but order some of the patients to do so.

For five days we were compelled to sit in the room all day. I never put in such a long time. Every patient was stiff and sore and tired. We would get in little groups on benches and torture our stomachs by conjuring up thoughts of what we would eat first when we got out. If I had not known how hungry they were and the pitiful side of it, the conversation would have been very amusing. As it was it only made me sad. When the subject of eating, which seemed to be the favorite one, was worn out, they used to give their opinions of the institution and its management. The condemnation of the nurses and the eatables was unanimous.

As the days passed Miss Tillie Mayard's condition grew worse. She was continually cold and unable to eat of the food provided. Day after day she sang in order to try to maintain her memory, but at last the nurse made her stop it. I talked with her daily, and I grieved to find her grow worse so rapidly. At last she got a delusion. She thought that I was trying to pass myself off for her, and that all the people who called to see Nellie Brown were friends in search of her, but that I, by some means, was trying to deceive them into the belief that I was the girl. I tried to reason with her, but found it impossible, so I kept away from her as much as possible, lest my presence should make her worse and feed the fancy.

One of the patients, Mrs. Cotter, a pretty, delicate woman, one day thought she saw her husband coming up the walk. She left the line in which she was marching and ran to meet him. For this act she was sent to the Retreat. She afterward said:

"The remembrance of that is enough to make me mad. For crying the nurses beat me with a broom-handle and jumped on me, injuring me internally, so that I shall never get over it. Then they tied my hands and feet, and, throwing a sheet over my head, twisted it tightly around my throat, so I could not scream, and thus put me in a bathtub filled with cold water. They held me under until I gave up every hope and became senseless. At other times they took hold of my ears and beat my head on the floor and against the wall. Then they pulled out my hair by the roots, so that it will never grow in again."

Mrs. Cotter here showed me proofs of her story, the dent in the back of her head and the bare spots where the hair had been taken out by the handful. I give her story as plainly as possible: "My treatment was not as bad as I have seen others get in there, but it has ruined my health, and even if I do get out of here I will be a wreck. When my husband heard of the treatment given me he threatened to expose the place if I was not removed, so I was brought here. I am well mentally now. All that old fear has left me, and the doctor has promised to allow my husband to take me home."

I made the acquaintance of Bridget McGuinness, who seems to be sane at the present time. She said she was sent to Retreat 4, and put on the "rope gang." "The beating I got there were something dreadful. I was pulled around by the hair, held under the water until I strangled, and I was choked and kicked. The nurses would always keep a quiet patient stationed at the window to tell them when any of the doctors were approaching. It was hopeless to complain to the doctors, for they always said it was the imagination of our diseased brains, and besides we would get another beating for telling. They would hold patients under the water and threaten to leave them to die there if they did not promise not to tell the doctors. We would all promise, because we knew the doctors would not help us, and we would do anything to escape the punishment. After breaking a window I was transferred to the Lodge, the worst place on the island. It is dreadfully dirty in there, and the stench is awful. In the summer the flies swarm the place. The food is worse than we get in other wards and we are given only tin plates. Instead of the bars being on the outside, as in this ward, they are on the inside. There are many quiet patients there who have been there for years, but the nurses keep them to do the work. Among other beating I got there, the nurses jumped on me once and broke two of my ribs.

"While I was there a pretty young girl was brought in. She had been sick, and she fought against being put in that dirty place. One night the nurses took her and, after beating her, they held her naked in a cold bath, then they threw her on her bed. When morning came the girl was dead. The doctors said she died of convulsions, and that was all that was done about it.

"They inject so much morphine and chloral that the patients are made crazy. I have seen the patients wild for water from the effect of the drugs, and the nurses would refuse it to them. I have heard women beg for a whole night for one drop and it was not given them. I myself cried for water until my mouth was so parched and dry that I could not speak."

I saw the same thing myself in hall 7. The patients would beg for a drink before retiring, but the nurses–Miss Hart and the others–refused to unlock the bathroom that they might quench their thirst.

CHAPTER XV.
INCIDENTS OF ASYLUM LIFE.

THERE is little in the wards to help one pass the time. All the asylum clothing is made by the patients, but sewing does not employ one's mind. After several months' confinement the thoughts of the busy world grow faint, and all the poor prisoners can do is to sit and ponder over their hopeless fate. In the upper halls a good view is obtained of the passing boats and New York. Often I tried to picture to myself as I looked out between the bars to the lights faintly glimmering in the city, what my feelings would be if I had no one to obtain my release.

I have watched patients stand and gaze longingly toward the city they in all likelihood will never enter again. It means liberty and life; it seems so near, and yet heaven is not further from hell.

Do the women pine for home? Excepting the most violent cases, they are conscious that they are confined in an asylum. An only desire that never dies is the one for release, for home.

One poor girl used to tell me every morning, "I dreamed of my mother last night. I think she may come to-day and take me home." That one thought, that longing, is always present, yet she has been confined some four years.

What a mysterious thing madness is. I have watched patients whose lips are forever sealed in a perpetual silence. They live, breathe, eat; the human form is there, but that something, which the body can live without, but which cannot exist without the body, was missing. I have wondered if behind those sealed lips there were dreams we ken not of, or if all was blank?

Still, as sad are those cases when the patients are always conversing with invisible parties. I have seen them wholly unconscious of their surroundings and engrossed with an invisible being. Yet, strange to say, that any command issued to them is always obeyed, in about the same manner as a dog obeys his master. One of the most pitiful delusions of any of the patients was that of a blue-eyed Irish girl, who believed she was forever damned because of one act in her life. Her horrible cry, morning and night, "I am damned for all eternity!" would strike horror to my soul. Her agony seemed like a glimpse of the inferno.

After being transferred to hall 7 I was locked in a room every night with six crazy women. Two of them seemed never to sleep, but spent the night in raving. One would get out of her bed and creep around the room searching for some one she wanted to kill. I could not help but think how easy it would be for her to attack any of the other patients confined with her. It did not make the night more comfortable.

One middle-aged woman, who used to sit always in the corner of the room, was very strangely affected. She had a piece of newspaper, and from it she continually read the most wonderful things I ever heard. I often sat close by her and listened. History and romance fell equally well from her lips.

I saw but one letter given a patient while I was there. It awakened a big interest. Every patient seemed thirsty for a word from the world, and they crowded around the one who had been so fortunate and asked hundreds of questions.

Visitors make but little interest and a great deal of mirth. Miss Mattie Morgan, in hall 7, played for the entertainment of some visitors one day. They were close about her until one whispered that she was a patient. "Crazy!" they whispered, audibly, as they fell back and left her alone. She was amused as well as indignant over the episode. Miss Mattie, assisted by several girls she has trained, makes the evenings pass very pleasantly in hall 7. They sing and dance. Often the doctors come up and dance with the patients.

One day when we went down to dinner we heard a weak little cry in the basement. Every one seemed to notice it, and it was not long until we knew there was a baby down there. Yes, a baby. Think of it–a little, innocent babe born in such a chamber of horrors! I can imagine nothing more terrible.

A visitor who came one day brought in her arms her babe. A mother who had been separated from her five little children asked permission to hold it. When the visitor wanted to leave, the woman's grief was uncontrollable, as she begged to keep the babe which she imagined was her own. It excited more patients than I had ever seen excited before at one time.

The only amusement, if so it may be called, given the patients outside, is a ride once a week, if the weather permits, on the "merry-go-round." It is a change, and so they accept it with some show of pleasure.

A scrub-brush factory, a mat factory, and the laundry, are where the mild patients work. They get no recompense for it, but they get hungry over it.

CHAPTER XVI.
THE LAST GOOD-BYE.

THE day Pauline Moser was brought to the asylum we heard the most horrible screams, and an Irish girl, only partly dressed, came staggering like a drunken person up the hall, yelling, "Hurrah! Three cheers! I have killed the divil! Lucifer, Lucifer, Lucifer," and so on, over and over again. Then she would pull a handful of hair out, while she exultingly cried, "How I deceived the divils. They always said God made hell, but he didn't." Pauline helped the girl to make the place hideous by singing the most horrible songs. After the Irish girl had been there an hour or so, Dr. Dent came in, and as he walked down the hall, Miss Grupe whispered to the demented girl, "Here is the devil coming, go for him." Surprised that she would give a mad woman such instructions, I fully expected to see the frenzied creature rush at the doctor. Luckily she did not, but commenced to repeat her refrain of "Oh, Lucifer." After the doctor left, Miss Grupe again tried to excite the woman by saying the pictured minstrel on the wall was the devil, and the poor creature began to scream, "You divil, I'll give it to you," so that two nurses had to sit on her to keep her down. The attendants seemed to find amusement and pleasure in exciting the violent patients to do their worst.

I always made a point of telling the doctors I was sane and asking to be released, but the more I endeavored to assure them of my sanity the more they doubted it.

"What are you doctors here for?" I asked one, whose name I cannot recall.

"To take care of the patients and test their sanity," he replied.

"Very well," I said. "There are sixteen doctors on this island, and excepting two, I have never seen them pay any attention to the patients. How can a doctor judge a woman's sanity by merely bidding her good morning and refusing to hear her pleas for release? Even the sick ones know it is useless to say anything, for the answer will be that it is their imagination." "Try every test on me," I have urged others, "and tell me am I sane or insane? Try my pulse, my heart, my eyes; ask me to stretch out my arm, to work my fingers, as Dr. Field did at Bellevue, and then tell me if I am sane." They would not heed me, for they thought I raved.

Again I said to one, "You have no right to keep sane people here. I am sane, have always been so and I must insist on a thorough examination or be released. Several of the women here are also sane. Why can't they be free?"

"They are insane," was the reply, "and suffering from delusions."

After a long talk with Dr. Ingram, he said, "I will transfer you to a quieter ward." An hour later Miss Grady called me into the hall, and, after calling me all the vile and profane names a woman could ever remember, she told me that it was a lucky thing for my "hide" that I was transferred, or else she would pay me for remembering so well to tell Dr. Ingram everything. "You d—n hussy, you forget all about yourself, but you never forget anything to tell the doctor." After calling Miss Neville, whom Dr. Ingram also kindly transferred, Miss Grady took us to the hall above, No. 7.

INSANE HALL NO. 7.

In hall 7 there are Mrs. Kroener, Miss Fitzpatrick, Miss Finney, and Miss Hart. I did not see as cruel treatment as down-stairs, but I heard them make ugly remarks and threats, twist the fingers and slap the faces of the unruly patients. The night nurse, Conway I believe her name is, is very cross. In hall 7, if any of the patients possessed any modesty, they soon lost it. Every one was compelled to undress in the hall before their own door, and to fold their clothes and leave them there until morning. I asked to undress in my room, but Miss Conway told me if she ever caught me at such a trick she would give me cause not to want to repeat it.

The first doctor I saw here–Dr. Caldwell–chucked me under the chin, and as I was tired refusing to tell where my home was, I would only speak to him in Spanish.

Hall 7 looks rather nice to a casual visitor. It is hung with cheap pictures and has a piano, which is presided over by Miss Mattie Morgan, who formerly was in a music store in this city. She has been training several of the patients to sing, with some show of success. The artiste of the hall is Under, pronounced Wanda, a Polish girl. She is a gifted pianist when she chooses to display her ability. The most difficult music she reads at a glance, and her touch and expression are perfect.

On Sunday the quieter patients, whose names have been handed in by the attendants during the week, are allowed to go to church. A small Catholic chapel is on the island, and other services are also held.

A "commissioner" came one day, and made the rounds with Dr. Dent. In the basement they found half the nurses gone to dinner, leaving the other half in charge of us, as was always done. Immediately orders were given to bring the nurses back to their duties until after the patients had finished eating. Some of the patients wanted to speak about their having no salt, but were prevented.

The insane asylum on Blackwell's Island is a human rat-trap. It is easy to get in, but once there it is impossible to get out. I had intended to have myself committed to the violent wards, the Lodge and Retreat, but when I got the testimony of two sane women and could give it, I decided not to risk my health—and hair—so I did not get violent.

I had, toward the last, been shut off from all visitors, and so when the lawyer, Peter A. Hendricks, came and told me that friends of mine were willing to take charge of me if I would rather be with them than in the asylum, I was only too glad to give my consent. I asked him to send me something to eat immediately on his arrival in the city, and then I waited anxiously for my release.

It came sooner than I had hoped. I was out "in line" taking a walk, and had just gotten interested in a poor woman who had fainted away while the nurses were trying to compel her to walk. "Good-bye; I am going home," I called to Pauline Moser, as she went past with a woman on either side of her. Sadly I said farewell to all I knew as I passed them on my way to freedom and life, while they were left behind to a fate worse than death. "*Adios*," I murmured to the Mexican woman. I kissed my fingers to her, and so I left my companions of hall 7.

I had looked forward so eagerly to leaving the horrible place, yet when my release came and I knew that God's sunlight was to be free for me again, there was a certain pain in leaving. For ten days I had been one of them. Foolishly enough, it seemed intensely selfish to leave them to their sufferings. I felt a Quixotic desire to help them by sympathy and presence. But only for a moment. The bars were down and freedom was sweeter to me than ever.

Soon I was crossing the river and nearing New York. Once again I was a free girl after ten days in the mad-house on Blackwell's Island.

CHAPTER XVII.
THE GRAND JURY INVESTIGATION.

SOON after I had bidden farewell to the Blackwell's Island Insane Asylum, I was summoned to appear before the Grand Jury. I answered the summons with pleasure, because I longed to help those of God's most unfortunate children whom I had left prisoners behind me. If I could not bring them that boon of all boons, liberty, I hoped at least to influence others to make life more bearable for them. I found the jurors to be gentlemen, and that I need not tremble before their twenty-three august presences.

I swore to the truth of my story, and then I related all–from my start at the Temporary Home until my release. Assistant District-Attorney Vernon M. Davis conducted the examination. The jurors then requested that I should accompany them on a visit to the Island. I was glad to consent.

No one was expected to know of the contemplated trip to the Island, yet we had not been there very long before one of the commissioners of charity and Dr. MacDonald, of Ward's Island, were with us. One of the jurors told me that in conversation with a man about the asylum, he heard that they were notified of our coming an hour before we reached the Island. This must have been done while the Grand Jury were examining the insane pavilion at Bellevue.

The trip to the island was vastly different to my first. This time we went on a clean new boat, while the one I had traveled in, they said, was laid up for repairs.

Some of the nurses were examined by the jury, and made contradictory statements to one another, as well as to my story. They confessed that the jury's contemplated visit had been talked over between them and the doctor. Dr. Dent confessed that he had no means by which to tell positively if the bath was cold and of the number of women put into the same water. He knew the food was not what it should be, but said it was due to the lack of funds.

If nurses were cruel to their patients, had he any positive means of ascertaining it? No, he had not. He said all the doctors were not competent, which was also due to the lack of means to secure good medical men. In the conversation with me, he said:

"I am glad you did this now, and had I known your purpose, I would have aided you. We have no means of learning the way things are going except to do as you did. Since your story was published I found a nurse at the Retreat who had watches set for our approach, just as you had stated. She was dismissed."

Miss Anne Neville was brought down, and I went into the hall to meet her, knowing that the sight of so many strange gentlemen would excite her, even if she be sane. It was as I feared. The attendants had told her she was going to be examined by a crowd of men, and she was shaking with fear. Although I had left her only two weeks before, yet she looked as if she had suffered a severe illness, in that time, so changed was her appearance. I asked her if she had taken any medicine, and she answered in the affirmative. I then told her that all I wanted her to do was tell the jury all we had done since I was brought with her to the asylum, so they would be convinced that I was sane. She only knew me as Miss Nellie Brown, and was wholly ignorant of my story.

She was not sworn, but her story must have convinced all hearers of the truth of my statements.

"When Miss Brown and I were brought here the nurses were cruel and the food was too bad to eat. We did not have enough clothing, and Miss Brown asked for more all the time. I thought she was very kind, for when a doctor promised her some clothing she said she would give it to me. Strange to say, ever since Miss Brown has been taken away everything is different. The nurses are very kind and we are given plenty to wear. The doctors come to see us often and the food is greatly improved."

Did we need more evidence?

The jurors then visited the kitchen. It was very clean, and two barrels of salt stood conspicuously open near the door! The bread on exhibition was beautifully white and wholly unlike what was given us to eat.

We found the halls in the finest order. The beds were improved, and in hall 7 the buckets in which we were compelled to wash had been replaced by bright new basins.

The institution was on exhibition, and no fault could be found.

But the women I had spoken of, where were they? Not one was to be found where I had left them. If my assertions were not true in regard to these patients, why should the latter be changed, so to make me unable to find them? Miss Neville complained before the jury of being changed several times. When we visited the hall later she was returned to her old place.

Mary Hughes, of whom I had spoken as appearing sane, was not to be found. Some relatives had taken her away. Where, they knew not. The fair woman I spoke of, who had been sent here because she was poor, they said had been transferred to another island. They denied all knowledge of the Mexican woman, and said there never had been such a patient. Mrs. Cotter had been discharged, and Bridget McGuinness and Rebecca Farron had been transferred to other quarters. The German girl, Margaret, was not to be found, and Louise had been sent elsewhere from hall 6. The Frenchwoman, Josephine, a great, healthy woman, they said was dying of paralysis, and we could not see her. If I was wrong in my judgment of these patients' sanity, why was all this done? I saw Tillie Mayard, and she had changed so much for the worse that I shuddered when I looked at her.

I hardly expected the grand jury to sustain me, after they saw everything different from what it had been while I was there. Yet they did, and their report to the court advises all the changes made that I had proposed.

I have one consolation for my work–on the strength of my story the committee of appropriation provides $1,000,000 more than was ever before given, for the benefit of the insane.

[THE END.]

New York City

Asylum for the Insane (Women)

Blackwell's Island

Miscellaneous Sketches.

BY NELLIE BLY.

TRYING TO BE A SERVANT.

MY STRANGE EXPERIENCE AT TWO EMPLOYMENT AGENCIES.

NONE but the initiated know what a great question the servant question is and how many perplexing sides it has. The mistresses and servants, of course, fill the leading *roles*. Then, in the lesser, but still important parts, come the agencies, which despite the many voices clamoring against them, declare themselves public benefactors. Even the "funny man" manages to fill a great deal of space with the subject. It is a serious question, since it affects all one holds dear in life–one's dinner, one's bed, and one's linen. I had heard so many complaints from long-suffering mistresses, worked-out servants, agencies, and lawyers, that I determined to investigate the subject to my own satisfaction. There was only one way to do it. That was to personate a servant and apply for a situation. I knew that there might be such things as "references" required, and, as I had never tested my abilities in this line, I did not know how to furnish them. Still, it would not do to allow a little thing like a "reference " to stop me in my work, and I would not ask any friend to commit herself to further my efforts. Many girls must at one time be without references, I thought, and this encouraged me to make the risk.

On Monday afternoon a letter came to the *World* office from a lawyer, complaining of an agency where, he claimed, a client of his had paid for a servant, and the agent then refused to produce a girl. This shop I decided to make my first essay. Dressed to look the character I wanted to represent, I walked up Fourth Avenue until I found No. 69, the place I wanted. It was a low frame building which retained all the impressions of old age. The room on the first floor was filled with a conglomeration of articles which gave it the appearance of a second-hand store. By a side door, leaning against the wall, was a large sign which told the passing public that that was the entrance to the "Germania Servants' Agency." On a straight, blue board, fastened lengthwise to a second-story window, was, in large, encouraging white letters, the ominous word "Servants."

I entered the side door, and as there was nothing before me but the dirty, uncarpeted hall and a narrow, rickety-looking staircase, I went on to my fate. I passed two closed doors on the first landing, and on the third I saw the word "Office." I did not knock, but turned the knob of the door, and, as it stuck top and bottom, I pressed my shoulder against it. It gave way, so did I, and I entered on my career as a servant with a tumble. It was a small room, with a low ceiling, a dusty ingrain carpet and cheaply papered walls. A heavy railing and a high desk and counter which divided the room gave it the appearance of a police court. Around the walls were hung colored advertisements of steamship lines and maps. Above the mantel, which was decorated with two plaster-paris busts, was a square sheet of white paper. I viewed the large black letters on this paper with a quaking heart. "References Investigated!!" with two exclamation points. Now, if it had only been put quietly and mildly, or even with one exclamation point, but two–dreadful. It was a death warrant to the idea I had of writing my own references if any were demanded.

IN THE INTELLIGENCE OFFICE.

A young woman who was standing with a downcast head by the window turned to look at the abrupt newcomer. A man who had apparently been conversing with her came hastily forward to the desk. He was a middle-sized man, with a sharp, gray eye, a bald head, and a black frock-coat buttoned up tightly, showing to disadvantage his rounded shoulders.

"Well?" he said to me, in a questioning manner, as he glanced quickly over my "get up."

"Are you the man who gets places for girls?" I asked, as if there were but one such man.

"Yes, I'm the man. Do you want a place?" he asked, with a decidedly German twang.

"Yes, I want a place," I replied.

"What did you work at last?"

"Oh, I was a chambermaid. Can you get me a position, do you think?"

"Yes, I can do that," he replied. "You're a nice-looking girl and I can soon get you a place. Just the other day I got a girl a place for $20 a month, just because she was nice-looking. Many gentlemen, and ladies also, will pay more when girls are nice-looking. Where did you work last?"

"I worked in Atlantic City," I replied, with a mental cry for forgiveness.

"Have you no city references?"

"No, none whatever; but I want a job in this city, that's why I came here."

"Well, I can get you a position, never fear, only some people are mighty particular about references."

"Have you no place you can send me to now?" I said, determined to get at my business as soon as possible.

"You have to pay to get your name entered on the book first," he said, opening a large ledger as he asked, "What is your name?"

"How much do you charge?" I asked, in order to give me time to decide on a name.

"I charge you one dollar for the use of the bureau for a month, and if I get you a big salary you will have to pay more."

"How much more?"

"That depends entirely on your salary," he answered, non-committal. "Your name?"

"Now, if I give you a dollar you will assure me a situation?"

"Certainly, that's what I'm here for."

"And you guarantee me work in this city?" I urged.

"Oh, certainly, certainly; that's what this agency is for. I'll get you a place, sure enough."

"All right, I'll give you a dollar, which is a great deal for a girl out of work. My name is Sally Lees."

"What shall I put you down for?" he asked.

OUT OF WORK.

"Oh, anything," I replied, with a generosity that surprised myself.

"Then I shall put it chambermaid, waitress, nurse or seamstress." So my name, or the one assumed, was entered in the ledger, and as I paid my dollar I ventured the information that if he gave me a situation directly I should be pleased to give him more money. He warmed up at this and told me he should advertise me in the morning.

"Then you have no one in want of help now?"

"We have plenty of people, but not just now. They all come in the morning. This is too late in the day. Where are you boarding?"

At this moment a woman clad in a blue dress, with a small, black shawl wrapped around her, entered from a room in the rear. She also looked me over sharply, as if I was an article for sale, as the man told her in German all that he knew about me.

"You can stay here," she said, in broken, badly broken English, after she had learned that I was friendless in the city. "Where is your baggage?"

"I left my baggage where I paid for my lodging to-night," I answered. They tried to induce me to stop at their house. Only $2.50 a week, with board, or 20 cents a night for a bed. They urged that it was immaterial to them, only I had a better chance to secure work if I was always there; it was only for my own good they suggested it. I had one glance of the adjoining bedroom, and that sight made me firm in my determination to sleep elsewhere.

As the evening drew on I felt they would have no more applications for servants that afternoon, and after asking the hour that I should return in the morning, I requested a receipt for my money. "You don't need to be so particular," he said, crossly, but I told him I was, and insisted until he was forced to comply. It was not much of a receipt. He wrote on the blank side of the agency's advertising card:

"Sally Lees has paid $1. Good for one month use of bureau. 69 4th Ave."

On the following morning, about 10:30, I made my appearance at the agency. Some eight or ten girls were in the room and the man who had pocketed my fee on the previous afternoon still adorned the throne back of the desk. No one said good-morning, or anything else for that matter, so I quietly slid onto a chair near the door. The girls were all comfortably dressed, and looked as if they had enjoyed hearty breakfasts. All sat silent, with a dreamy expression on their faces, except two who stood by the window watching the passing throng and conversing in whispers with one another. I wanted to be with or near them, so that I might hear what was said. After waiting for some time I decided to awake the man to the fact that I wanted work, not a rest.

"Have you no place to send me this morning?"

"No; but I advertised you in the paper," and he handed me the *Tribune* of October 25 and pointed out the following notice:

"NURSE,&c.–By excellent, very neat English girl as nurse and seamstress, chambermaid and waitress, or parlor maid. Call at 69 4th ave.; no cards answered."

I choked down a laugh as I read myself advertised in this manner, and wondered what my *role* would be the next time. I began to hope some one would soon call for the excellent girl, but when an aged gentleman entered I wished just as fervently that he was not after me. I was enjoying my position too much, and I fear I could not restrain my gravity if any one began to question me. Poor old gentleman! He looked around helplessly, as if he was at a loss to know what to do. The agent did not leave him long in doubt. "You want a girl, sir?"

"Yes, my wife read an advertisement in the *Tribune* this morning, and she sent me here to see the girl."

"Yes, yes, excellent girl, sir, come right back here," opening the gates and giving the gentleman a chair behind the high counter. "You come here, Sally Lees," indicating a chair beside the visitor for me. I sat down with an inward chuckle and the agent leaned over the back of a chair. The visitor eyed me nervously, and after clearing his throat several times and making vain attempts at a beginning, he said:

"You are the girl who wants work?" And after I answered in the affirmative, he said: "Of course you know how to do all these things–you know what is required of a girl?"

"Oh, yes, I know," I answered confidently.

"Yes–well, how much do you want a month?"

"Oh, anything," I answered, looking to the agent for aid. He understood the look, for he began hurriedly:

"Fourteen dollars a month, sir. She is an excellent girl, good, neat, quick and of an amiable disposition."

I was astonished at his knowledge of my good qualities, but I maintained a lofty silence.

"Yes, yes," the visitor said, musingly. "My wife only pays ten dollars a month, and then if the girl is all right she is willing to pay more, you know. I really couldn't, you know—"

"We have no ten-dollar-girls here, sir," said the agent with dignity; "you can't get an honest, neat, and respectable girl for that amount."

"H'm, yes; well, this girl has good references, I suppose?"

94

"Oh, yes; I know all about her," said the agent, briskly and confidently. "She is an excellent girl, and I can give you the best personal reference– the best of references."

Here I was, unknown to the agent. So far as he knew, I might be a confidence woman, a thief, or everything wicked, and yet the agent was vowing that he had good personal references.

"Well, I live in Bloomfield, N.J., and there are only four in the family. Of course you are a good washer and ironer?" he said, turning to me. Before I had time to assure him of my wonderful skill in that line, the agent interposed: "This is not the girl you want. No, sir, this girl won't do general housework. This is the girl you are after," bringing up another. "She does general housework," and he went on with a long list of her virtues, which were similar to those he had professed to find in me. The visitor got very nervous and began to insist that he could not take a girl unless his wife saw her first. Then the agent, when he found it impossible to make him take a girl, tried to induce the gentleman to join the bureau. "It will only cost you $2 for the use of the bureau for a month," he urged, but the visitor began to get more nervous and to make his way to the door. I thought he was frightened because it was an agency, and it amused me to hear how earnestly he pleaded that really he dare not employ a girl without his wife's consent.

After the escape of this visitor we all resumed our former positions and waited for another visitor. It came in the shape of a red-haired Irish girl.

"Well, you are back again?" was the greeting given her.

"Yes. That woman was horrible. She and her husband fought all the time, and the cook carried tales to the mistress. Sure and I wouldn't live at such a place. A splendid laundress, with a good 'karacter,' don't need to stay in such places, I told them. The lady of the house made me wash every other day; then she wanted me to be dressed like a lady, sure, and wear a cap while I was at work. Sure and it's no good laundress who can be dressed up while at work, so I left her."

The storm had scarcely passed when another girl with fiery locks entered. She had a good face and a bright one, and I watched her closely.

95

"So you are back, too. You are troublesome," said the agent. Her eyes flashed as she replied:

"Oh, I'm troublesome, am I? Well, you can take a poor girl's money, anyway, and then you tell her she's troublesome. It wasn't troublesome when you took my money; and where is the position? I have walked all over the city, wearing out my shoes and spending my money in car-fare. Now, is this how you treat poor girls?"

"I did not mean anything by saying you were troublesome. That was only my fun," the agent tried to explain; and after awhile the girl quieted down.

Another girl came and was told that as she had not made her appearance the day previous she could not expect to obtain a situation. He refused to send her word if there was any chance. Then a messenger boy called and said that Mrs. Vanderpool, of No. 36 West Thirty-ninth Street, wanted the girl advertised in the morning paper. Irish girl No. 1 was sent, and she returned, after several hours' absence, to say that Mrs. Vanderpool said, when she learned where the girl came from, that she knew all about agencies and their schemes, and she did not propose to have a girl from them. The girl buttoned Mrs. Vanderpool's shoes, and returned to the agency to take her post of waiting.

I succeeded at last in drawing one of the girls, Winifred Friel, into conversation. She said she had been waiting for several days, and that she had no chance of a place yet. The agency had a place out of town to which they tried to force girls who declared they would not leave the city. Quite strange they never offered the place to girls who said they would work anywhere. Winifred Friel wanted it, but they would not allow her to go, yet they tried to insist on me accepting it.

"Well, now, if you won't take that I would like to see you get a place this winter," he said, angrily, when he found that I would not go out of the city.

"Why, you promised that you would find me a situation in the city."

"That's no difference; if you won't take what I offer you can do without," he said indifferently.

"Then give me my money," I said.

"No, you can't have your money. That goes into the bureau." I urged and insisted, to no avail, and so I left the agency, to return no more.

My second day I decided to apply to another agency, so I went to Mrs. L. Seely's, No. 68 Twenty-second Street. I paid my dollar fee and was taken to the third story and put in a small room which was packed as close with women as sardines in a box. After edging my way in I was unable to move, so packed were we. A woman came up, and, calling me "that tall girl," told me roughly as I was new it was useless for me to wait there. Some of the girls said Mrs. Seely was always cross to them, and that I should not mind it. How horribly stifling those rooms were! There were fifty-two in the room with me, and the two other rooms I could look into were equally crowded, while groups stood on the stairs and in the hallway. It was a novel insight I got of life. Some girls laughed, others were sad, some slept, some ate, and others read, while all sat from morning till night waiting a chance to earn a living. They are long waits too. One girl had been there two months, others for days and weeks. It was good to see the glad look when called out to see a lady, and sad to see them return saying that they did not suit because they wore bangs, or their hair in the wrong style, or that they looked bilious, or that they were too tall, too short, too heavy, or too slender. One poor woman could not obtain a place because she wore mourning, and so the objections ran.

I got no chance the entire day, and I decided that I could not endure a second day in that human pack for two situations, so framing some sort of excuse I left the place, and gave up trying to be a servant.

Nellie Bly as a White Slave.

HER EXPERIENCE IN THE ROLE OF A NEW YORK SHOP-GIRL MAKING PAPER BOXES.

ERY early the other morning I started out, not with the pleasure-seekers, but with those who toil the day long that they may live. Everybody was rushing–girls of all ages and appearances and hurrying men–and I went along, as one of the throng. I had often wondered at the tales of poor pay and cruel treatment that working girls tell. There was one way of getting at the truth, and I determined to try it. It was becoming myself a paper box factory girl. Accordingly, I started out in search of work without experience, reference, or aught to aid me.

It was a tiresome search, to say the least. Had my living depended on it, it would have been discouraging, almost maddening. I went to a great number of factories in and around Bleecker and Grand streets and Sixth Avenue, where the workers number up into the hundreds. "Do you know how to do the work?" was the question asked by every one. When I replied that I did not, they gave me no further attention.

"I am willing to work for nothing until I learn," I urged.

"Work for nothing! Why, if you paid us for coming we wouldn't have you in our way," said one.

"We don't run an establishment to teach women trades," said another, in answer to my plea for work.

"Well, as they are not born with the knowledge, how do they ever learn?" I asked.

THE PASTING TABLE.

"The girls always have some friend who wants to learn. If she wishes to lose time and money by teaching her, we don't object, for we get the work the beginner does for nothing."

By no persuasion could I obtain an entree into the larger factories, so I concluded at last to try a smaller one at No. 196 Elm Street. Quite unlike the unkind, brusque men I had met at other factories, the man here was very polite. He said: "If you have never done the work, I don't think you will like it. It is dirty work and a girl has to spend years at it before she can make much money. Our beginners are girls about sixteen years old, and they do not get paid for two weeks after they come here."

"What can they make afterward?"

"We sometimes start them at week work–$1.50 a week. When they become competent they go on piecework–that is, they are paid by the hundred."

"How much do they earn then?"

"A good worker will earn from $5 to $9 a week."

"Have you many girls here?"

"We have about sixty in the building and a number who take work home. I have only been in this business for a few months, but if you think you would like to try it, I shall speak to my partner. He has had some of his girls for eleven years. Sit down until I find him."

He left the office, and I soon heard him talking outside about me, and rather urging that I be given a chance. He soon returned, and with him a small man who spoke with a German accent. He stood by me without speaking, so I repeated by request. "Well, give your name to the gentleman at the desk, and come down on Monday morning, and we will see what we can do for you."

And so it was that I started out early in the morning. I had put on a calico dress to work in and to suit my chosen trade. In a nice little bundle, covered with brown paper with a grease-spot on the center of it, was my lunch. I had an idea that every working girl carried a lunch, and I was trying to give out the impression that I was quite used to this thing. Indeed, I considered the lunch a telling stroke of thoughtfulness in my new *role*, and eyed with some pride, in which was mixed a little dismay, the grease-spot, which was gradually growing in size.

Early as it was I found all the girls there and at work. I went through a small wagon-yard, the only entrance to the office. After making my excuses to the gentleman at the desk, he called to a pretty little girl, who had her apron full of pasteboard, and said:

"Take this lady up to Norah."

"Is she to work on boxes or cornucopias?" asked the girl.

"Tell Norah to put her on boxes."

Following my little guide, I climbed the narrowest, darkest, and most perpendicular stair it has ever been my misfortune to see. On and on we went, through small rooms, filled with working girls, to the top floor–fourth or fifth story, I have forgotten which. Any way, I was breathless when I got there.

"Norah, here is a lady you are to put on boxes," called out my pretty little guide.

All the girls that surrounded the long tables turned from their work and looked at me curiously. The auburn-haired girl addressed as Norah raised her eyes from the box she was making, and replied:

"See if the hatchway is down, and show her where to put her clothes."

Then the forewoman ordered one of the girls to "get the lady a stool," and sat down before a long table, on which was piled a lot of pasteboard squares, labeled in the center. Norah spread some long slips of paper on the table; then taking up a scrub-brush, she dipped it into a bucket of paste and then rubbed it over the paper. Next she took one of the squares of pasteboard and, running her thumb deftly along, turned up the edges. This done, she took one of the slips of paper and put it quickly and neatly over the corner, binding them together and holding them in place. She quickly cut the paper off at the edge with her thumb-nail and swung the thing around and did the next corner. This I soon found made a box lid. It looked and was very easy, and in a few moments I was able to make one.

I did not find the work difficult to learn, but rather disagreeable. The room was not ventilated, and the paste and glue were very offensive. The piles of boxes made conversation impossible with all the girls except a beginner, Therese, who sat by my side. She was very timid at first, but after I questioned her kindly she grew more communicative.

"I live on Eldrige Street with my parents. My father is a musician, but he will not go on the streets to play. He very seldom gets an engagement. My mother is sick nearly all the time. I have a sister who works at passementerie. She can earn from $3 to $5 a week. I have another sister who has been spooling silk in Twenty-third Street for five years now. She makes $6 a week. When she comes home at night her face and hands and hair are all colored from the silk she works on during the day. It makes her sick, and she is always taking medicine."

"Have you worked before?"

"Oh, yes; I used to work at passementerie on Spring Street. I worked from 7 until 6 o'clock, piecework, and made about $3.50 a week. I left because the bosses were not kind, and we only had three little oil lamps to see to work by. The rooms were very dark, but they never allowed us to burn the gas. Ladies used to come here and take the work home to do. They did it cheap, for the pleasure of doing it, so we did not get as much pay as we would otherwise."

"What did you do after you left there?" I asked.

"I went to work in a fringe factory on Canal Street. A woman had the place and she was very unkind to all the girls. She did not speak English. I worked an entire week, from 8 to 6, with only a half-hour for dinner, and at the end of the week she only paid me 35 cents. You know a girl cannot live on 35 cents a week, so I left."

"How do you like the box factory?"

"Well, the bosses seem very kind. They always say good-morning to me, a thing never done in any other place I ever worked, but it is a good deal for a poor girl to give two weeks' work for nothing. I have been here almost two weeks, and I have done a great deal of work. It's all clear gain to the bosses. They say they often dismiss a girl after her first two weeks on the plea that she does not suit. After this I am to get $1.50 a week."

When the whistles of the surrounding factories blew at 12 o'clock the forewoman told us we could quit work and eat our lunch. I was not quite so proud of my cleverness in simulating a working girl when one of them said:

"Do you want to send out for your lunch?"

"No; I brought it with me," I replied.

"Oh!" she exclaimed, with a knowing inflection and amused smile.

"Is there anything wrong?" I asked, answering her smile.

FINISHING UP.

"Oh, no," quickly; "only the girls always make fun of any one who carries a basket now. No working-girl will carry a lunch or basket. It is out of style because it marks the girl at once as a worker. I would like to carry a basket, but I don't dare, because they would make so much fun of me."

The girls sent out for lunch and I asked of them the prices. For five cents they get a good pint of coffee, with sugar and milk if desired. Two cents will buy three slices of buttered bread. Three cents, a sandwich. Many times a number of the girls will put all their money together and buy quite a little food. A bowl of soup for five cents will give four girls a taste. By clubbing together they are able to buy warm lunch.

At one o'clock we were all at work again. I having completed sixty-four lids, and the supply being consumed was put at "molding in." This is fitting the bottom into the sides of the box and pasting it there. It is rather difficult at first to make all the edges come closely and neatly together, but after a little experience it can be done easily.

On my second day I was put at a table with some new girls and I tried to get them to talk. I was surprised to find that they are very timid about telling their names, where they live or how. I endeavored by every means a woman knows, to get an invitation to visit their homes, but did not succeed.

"How much can girls earn here?" I asked the forewoman.

"I do not know," she said; "they never tell each other, and the bosses keep their time."

"Have you worked here long?" I asked.

"Yes, I have been here eight years, and in that time I have taught my three sisters."

"Is the work profitable?"

"Well, it is steady; but a girl must have many years' experience before she can work fast enough to earn much."

The girls all seem happy. During the day they would make the little building resound with their singing. A song would be begun on the second floor, probably, and each floor would take it up in succession, until all were singing. They were nearly always kind to one another. Their little quarrels did not last long, nor were they very fierce. They were all extremely kind to me, and did all they could to make my work easy and pleasant. I felt quite proud when able to make an entire box.

There were two girls at one table on piecework who had been in a great many box factories and had had a varied experience.

"Girls do not get paid half enough at any work. Box factories are no worse than other places. I do not know anything a girl can do where by hard work she can earn more than $6 a week. A girl cannot dress and pay her boarding on that."

"Where do such girls live?" I asked.

"There are boarding-places on Bleecker and Houston, and around such places, where girls can get a room and meals for $3.50 a week. The room may be only for two, in one bed, or it may have a dozen, according to size. They have no conveniences or comforts, and generally undesirable men board at the same place."

"Why don't they live at these homes that are run to accommodate working women?"

"Oh, those homes are frauds. A girl cannot obtain any more home comforts, and then the restrictions are more than they will endure. A girl who works all day must have some recreation, and she never finds it in homes."

"Have you worked in box factories long?"

"For eleven years, and I can't say that it has ever given me a living. On an average I make $5 a week. I pay out $3.50 for board, and my wash bill at the least is 75 cents. Can any one expect a woman to dress on what remains?"

"What do you get paid for boxes?"

"I get 50 cents a hundred for one-pound candy boxes, and 40 cents a hundred for half-pound boxes."

"What work do you do on a box for that pay?"

"Everything. I get the pasteboard cut in squares the same as you did. I first 'set up' the lids, then I 'mold in' the bottoms. This forms a box. Next I do the 'trimming,' which is putting the gilt edge around the box lid. 'Cover striping' (covering the edge of the lid) is next, and then comes the 'top label,' which finishes the lid entire. Then I paper the box, do the 'bottom labeling,' and then put in two or four laces (lace paper) on the inside as ordered. Thus you see one box passes through my hands eight times before it is finished. I have to work very hard and without ceasing to be able to make two hundred boxes a day, which earns me $1. It is not enough pay. You see I handle two hundred boxes sixteen hundred times for $1. Cheap labor, isn't it?"

One very bright girl, Maggie, who sat opposite me, told a story that made my heart ache.

"This is my second week here," she said, "and, of course, I won't receive any pay until next week, when I expect to receive $1.50 for six days' work. My father was a driver before he got sick. I don't know what is wrong, but the doctor says he will die. Before I left this morning he said my father

105

will die soon. I could hardly work because of it. I am the oldest child, and I have a brother and two sisters younger. I am sixteen, and my brother is twelve. He gets $2 a week for being office-boy at a cigar-box factory."

"Do you have much rent to pay?"

"We have two rooms in a house on Houston Street. They are small and have low ceilings, and there are a great many Chinamen in the same house. We pay for these rooms $14 per month. We do not have much to eat, but then father doesn't mind it because he can't eat. We could not live if father's lodge did not pay our rent."

"Did you ever work before?"

"Yes, I once worked in a carpet factory at Yonkers. I only had to work there one week until I learned, and afterward I made at piecework a dollar a day. When my father got so ill my mother wanted me at home, but now when we see I can earn so little they wish I had remained there."

"Why do you not try something else?" I asked.

"I wanted to, but could find nothing. Father sent me to school until I was fourteen, and so I thought I would learn to be a telegraph operator. I went to a place in Twenty-third Street, where it is taught, but the man said he would not give me a lesson unless I paid fifty dollars in advance. I could not do that."

I then spoke of the Cooper Institute, which I thought every New Yorker knew was for the benefit of just such cases. I was greatly astonished to learn that such a thing as the Cooper Institute was wholly unknown to all the workers around me.

"If my father knew that there was a free school he would send me," said one.

"I would go in the evenings," said another, "if I had known there was such a place."

Again, when some of them were complaining of unjust wages, and some of places where they had been unable to collect the amount due them after

106

working, I spoke of the mission of the Knights of Labor, and the newly organized society for women. They were all surprised to hear that there were any means to aid women in having justice. I moralized somewhat on the use of any such societies unless they entered the heart of these factories.

One girl who worked on the floor below me said they were not allowed to tell what they earned. However, she had been working here five years, and she did not average more than $5 a week. The factory in itself was a totally unfit place for women. The rooms were small and there was no ventilation. If case of fire there was practically no escape.

The work was tiresome, and after I had learned all I could from the rather reticent girls I was anxious to leave. I noticed some rather peculiar things on my trip to and from the factory. I noticed that men were much quicker to offer their places to the working-girls on the cars than they were to offer them to well-dressed women. Another thing quite as noticeable, I had more men try to get up a flirtation with me while I was a box-factory girl than I ever had before. The girls were nice in their manners and as polite as ones reared at home. They never forgot to thank one another for the slightest service, and there was quite a little air of "good form" in many of their actions. I have seen many worse girls in much higher positions than the white slaves of New York.

THE END.

Other Writings by Nellie Bly.

NELLIE BLY IN JAIL By Nellie Bly

The New York World/January 20, 1895

Chats with Eugene Victor Debs, the Imprisoned Labor Leader

How He and Comrades Pass Time

They Lead Rather a Jolly Life Telling Stories, Reading and Enjoying Good Meals

Debs Glad That He is not Rich

He Would Rather Be an Orator than to Be a Millionaire,

For He Thinks the Wealthy Are Objects of Pity

Chicago, Ill., Jan, 18 – Eugene Victor Debs says he makes only one sacrifice by being in jail. That is the absence from his family circle in their Sunday evening reunions.

It has been the invariable custom of the Debs family to spend their Sunday evenings together. As children it was the unbroken rule and as the sons and daughters grew up and got homes of their own, they still came back on Sunday evenings with husbands or wives and children to their parents' fireside.

"All days are alike to one in jail," Mr. Debs said to me. "I forget whether it's Monday or Wednesday, but intuitively and without effort I know when it's Sunday. I suppose one would say it was due to some occult influence, for then the family are together and my chair is vacant."

While I attended the strikes at Pullman last summer I did not meet Mr. Debs, who as the leader of the A. R. U., became so widely known through them. So I was rather glad to take the tiresome trip to Woodstock, Ill., to see Mr. Debs.

Woodstock is a small country town. The jail is a very small affair in the rear of the Sheriff's house, and adjoining the court-house.

The reason Mr. Debs and his seven fellow-sufferers are in Woodstock is because the jail in Chicago is overflowing with prisoners, guilty and innocent, and, unlike the street cars, it cannot squeeze in another one. They have at present four men in every small cell, and the entire place is crawling with vermin and deep in filth. So Mr. Debs and his companions have good reasons for congratulating themselves that there was no room for more.

There are no signs of a jail about the front of the sheriff's house. It is a plain brick, with unbarred windows. I rang the bell, and was admitted by a young girl, who stared at me wonderingly.

"I would like to see Mr. Debs. Can I do so?" I asked.

"I guess so," she said, and then added, hesitatingly, "the Sheriff's in court and won't be out till 12, so I guess I'd better ask mother."

She disappeared after telling me to be seated, and presently a woman came in and I made known to her my wishes.

"Are you his wife?" she asked, curiously.

"No;" I replied, "merely a friend."

"I guess you can see him. Come this way," she said.

I followed her through the dining room to a hall in the rear and along this hall to where iron bars, newly painted white, shut off the jail from the house.

Glancing through the bars I could see a number of men sitting in a sun-lit corridor. They all sat in perfect silence, deeply interested in the books they are reading.

"Here's a friend of yours, Mr. Debs," the woman called, and Mr. Debs came close to the gate.

I did not want everybody to know who I was, so I whispered through the bars.

"I am Nellie Bly, Mr. Debs, and I would like to have a talk with you."

"I am glad to see you, Miss Bly," was the quiet reply, and then he addressed the woman.

"Can you let me come out for a little while, Mrs. Eckert?" he said.

"I'll let you out alone," she replied, and taking a huge key from her pocket endeavored to unlock the door.

The lock stuck.

"Push on the door, Mr. Debs," she ordered, and Mr. Debs lent his aid to undo the stubborn bolt.

His Own Jailer

"The other night I had to lock myself in," Mr. Debs observed dryly.

In another moment the bolt shot back, the door swung open and Eugene Victor Debs stood in the corridor before me.

For an instant we looked at each other, his tall figure looming up before me, and then simultaneously we stretched out our arms.

"I am glad to meet you," said Mr. Debs.

"And I am glad to meet you," I replied.

110

Side by side we walked through the corridor, through the dining-room and to the sitting-room which I had first entered.

There we sat down facing each other.

"They don't seem much afraid of your getting away," I observed.

"They know we are on our honor here, and they can trust us." Mr. Debs replied, "The day we were brought here I was to appear in court at 10 o'clock. I had been in St. Paul, and when I arrived in Chicago it was almost 10 o'clock, so I ran all the way to court and arrived there just one minute to 10. I was on my honor, and I would not have been a minute late for anything in the world. Several persons said to me that I was the first man they ever saw run to get into jail."

"Do you find your imprisonment very hard to bear?" I asked.

No, the only thing I miss is the separation from my family. It has always been the custom of our family to have a reunion Sunday nights, and to miss them is the only cross I have to bear. My father and mother are old, my father being seventy-five, and it is hard to miss even one night that I could be with them."

The Debs family is a very happy and lucky one. There are four daughters and two sons, and there has never been a death. The daughters married and the sons married, and it only increased the family circle. Even the very slightest of family quarrels or strife has never come among the Debses.

Eugene Victor Debs says the most perfect harmony and affection have always existed in his home, even with those who have married into his family.

He has been married ten years, and he has never had even one cross word with his wife.

She is a daughter, fond and loving, to his parents, and she is in the family circle these Sunday evenings that he spends in jail.

Until within a short time the family all lived in Terre Haute, Ind., but now one married sister lives in New York and another is on a visit to Paris, while Mr. Debs is in jail, making a break in the home that the parents feel deeply.

"Don't you think it is rather hard to be in jail on the silly charge of contempt of court, when Carnegie is at liberty?" I asked.

Mr. Debs smiled.

"Everybody understands what makes the difference." he answered. "You know," he added, "they declared me guilty under the bill known as the Interstate Commerce Law.

This bill was supposedly enacted for the protection of small farmers and producers. Before the law was passed the small farmers were crushed to the wall by combines and large companies, who could get low rates because of the quantity they shipped, and consequently were always able to undersell the small farmer.

"Since the Santa Fe Railroad has been in the hands of receivers, Expert Little, who made an examination of the company's books, finds that J. W. Reinhardt, president of the company, paid out, within a year, $8,000,000 in rebates to favored shippers, the very thing the Interstate Commerce Law was designed to put a stop to. No one was ever prosecuted. Mr. Reinhardt was permitted to resign his position, and the matter ended there.

Notwithstanding the Sante Fe Company was in the hands of a receiver, therefore in the custody of the court, the court took no judicial knowledge of the crime, and nothing has been said of it from that day to this. Had it been a labor leader guilty of this crime, the press would have insisted on his being prosecuted and published by fine and imprisonment, and there would have been no end until this was done."

Compared With Millionaires

I looked at Mr. Debs as he sat before me and compared him with two millionaires—Pullman and Carnegie.

Mr. Debs is unusually tall—an inch or two over six feet, I should judge. He is well built, slender, but not thin. His shoulders are broad and there is a look of strength about him.

His face is rather long, beardless and smooth cut. He has the strong, large nose of a successful man. His mouth is small and pleasantly shaped, and he smiles frequently, a fleeting but pretty smile that shows two rows of strong white teeth.

His eyes are blue, and at present have slightly reddish rings about them, as though from too much reading. Gold-rimmed glasses that run behind the ears he wears constantly.

Mr. Debs' forehead was originally high and broad, and much thought has placed four lines across it, with a short one above the right eye. There are evidences that in a short time Mr. Debs' forehead will be still higher. His hair is very thin on top.

There was no sign of the prisoner about Mr. Debs' clothes. He wore a well-made suit of gray tweed, the coat being a cutaway, and a white starched shirt with a standing collar and a small black and white scarf tied in a bow-knot.

There was a plain gold button in his shirt front, a gold chain crossing from buttonhole to vest pocket and an agate ring upon the third finger of his left hand.

"You don't seem very fond of jewelry," I observed.

"No; I've had a great deal given to me, but I do not like it....I only wear this ring, and I've worn it for fifteen years, for one reason. You can see why."

He took off the ring and handed it to me, and I saw inscribed on the inside—"Mother to Eugene."

Eugene Victor Debs' parents were born in France, but all their children were born in America. Mr. Debs, Sr., was a grocer in Terre Haute. His son, Eugene, was born Nov. 5, 1855, and attended the public schools until he was fourteen years old, when he went to work in the Vandalia Railroad paint shops.

For a year and a half he earned 50 cents a day, until ill-health forced him to stop.

113

Afterwards he "fired" on a locomotive for the same company for three years and a half. He was passionately fond of railroading, and might have been working at it yet had not a wreck occurred in which two of his comrades, the engineer and fireman, were killed. This affected his mother so strongly that she insisted upon his leaving the business.

So Eugene Debs left railroading for the grocery business. There is a wholesale grocery house in Terra Haute that is considered the most complete in America. In this the young man worked for five years, and held one of the most responsible positions in the house, when he became ambitious politically. He was successful in his first campaign, and in 1880 became city clerk. Five years later he was elected to the legislature.

This, he says, settled all his political aspirations. He saw that if he expected to accomplish anything he must adapt himself to the existing methods, and this he could not do and retain his self-respect.

Since 1876 Mr. Debs had been a member of the Brotherhood of Locomotive Firemen, and when, some four years later, the secretary was found to be a defaulter, the order being bankrupted and demoralized in consequence, Mr. Debs was called upon to fill the unexpired term.

Refused A Trip

This he did with great success, and in a short time had succeeded in paying off the debt of $8,000. After that he was appointed editor of the Locomotive Firemen's Magazine, and held that position until 1888. He resigned then, though unanimously re-elected, with the privilege of fixing his own salary. The order also voted him $3,000 and a six months' vacation, but Mr. Debs refused to take the money, and it still remains in the treasury of the Brotherhood.

Mr. Debs' reason for quitting the paper was that he might lend his aid to the order in other ways. He thought he had a mission to perform, and he set out to do it. He had recognized the fact that all the railroads were secretly coming together, and that they meant to reduce wages, not everywhere at once, but quietly, first one place and then another, until a wholesale reduction would result.

This is what Eugene Victor Debs wanted to work against. And if his records are anything, I don't know of any man who would make a better leader for any class of people. Eugene Debs has been in labor organizations for twenty years.

While success invariably creates enemies, and the most malicious of all enemies, failure also produces enemies, but Eugene Debs has never had a candidate named against him nor a vote cast against him in all these twenty years.

That says a great deal for the man.

In addition to this, it was plain to everybody that his motive must be an honest one, since he never tried to make money from his position, but on the contrary at every convention has always asked to have his salary reduced from one to two thousand dollars.

He gave up a yearly salary of $3,000 to work for the Railroad Union at $75 per month, and when the trouble broke out the convention voted to raise his salary to $3,000. But he decided the order needed the money, and he stopped his salary and has not received any since.

"How have you managed to live?" I asked, impertinently perhaps, but curiously.

"Through my family," he replied. "Whatever one has is for all. There is not a discord in our entire connection, and whatever the others have is at the command of any who may need it."

"Are you worth any money?" I asked.

"The extent of my worldly possessions is a house and lot," he answered. "I owe no man a dollar and no man owes me. You might say that I am square with the world."

"Have you no ambition to get rich?"

"Not the least. If I had to take my choice between being extremely rich or extremely poor, I would choose the later. I think the very rich deserve pity instead of censure, just as Oscar Wilde says in his latest essay we ought not to be severe with the very rich, they as well as the poor are entitled to

115

our commiseration. Money-getting is a disease as much as paresis, and as much to be pitied."

"What is your highest ambition?"

"All my life, from my earliest recollection, my highest ambition has been to be an orator," he answered, his earnest blue eyes looking steadily at me. "I have always thought the personality or power to move people was the greatest on earth. If I had my choice of the gifts that come to men, I would choose that. If a woman, I would want to be the most beautiful singer."

When Mr. Debs was "firing" he worked all night, slept in the forenoon and attended school in the afternoon. He has heard all the orators with any pretensions to greatness and power.

Fond Of Music

Mr. Debs is passionately fond of music. His wife and her sisters and his own are all musical. The piano, banjo, mandolin and guitar are all played in his house.

Mr. Debs understands French and speaks German. He doesn't care much for novels, except for those of Hugo, Sue and Dumas. Lately he reads only economic works.

He smokes, is temperate, but enjoys a good dinner and is fond of pets. He has two—Fay, an Irish setter, and a canary named "Sweetie."

He is passionately fond of children, and one can readily believe him when he says all the children at home know him.

He told me of a little incident that happened just before he left his home this last time, and which warmed his heart to endure the trial before him.

On the morning of the day he left there came a timid knock upon his door, and, opening it, he saw two little tots, a boy and a girl, on the step. Each carried a little red savings bank.

The little boy was spokesman.

"I got $13," he said, "and sister's got two in her bank, and we're going to give it to you to pay those men so they won't take you off to jail."

They had evidently heard their parents discussing Mr. Debs' fate and had made up their baby minds to save their favorite.

Mr. Debs has no children of his own.

There is much of a poetic nature in Eugene Debs. He has a soft pleasing voice, a voice that is soothing and caressing. His manner is most mild and gentle. For some reason which I cannot explain he reminds me of James Whitcomb Riley. He and Riley are warm personal friends.

"Riley says every man lives his life in a circle," he said to me during our conversation. "A man starts here (drawing an imaginary circle upon his knee), a farm lad. He drifts out to a city to make wealth, but after a while he tires of his money and the hurry and bustle of the world, and he buys a farm, and after a while his friends go out to see him and find him happy at work among his cattle, just where he began as a boy. So he completes his circle."

"I know how my life is to be," he continued, in a dreamy fashion, his blue eyes gazing out through the window, where everything glistened with snow. "I am going to die in perfect quiet on a farm. I know just what that farm is like, though I have never seen it. A winding creek cuts through it and there is an immense orchard."

He stopped suddenly as if he thought he was too confidential, and smiled, "You see," he explained, "I want a little poetry in it. I always considered a farmer's life should be the freest and best in the world. If any man knows liberty, it should be the farmer. If any man is wise, it should be the farmer. It is a perfect life. I never pass a farm-house that I do not envy the inmates. In the country one does as one likes: In the city one does as others like. The country is the only place a man can be true to himself."

In the lapel of his coat Mr. Debs wore a very brilliant pink. He evidently thought I noticed it.

"I suppose people might think this seems out of place—a carnation on a convict!" he observed with a merry smile, "and that I should wear weeping willow or something like that. It was among a box of flowers which the

117

wife of one of my comrades sent all the way from Ogden, Utah. They came in a beautiful condition: just as fresh as if newly out."

Mr. Debs is a class student of Shakespeare, and always carries a volume with him. He can repeat Romeo and Juliet and Julius Caesar almost entire.

He is getting pretty well used to the newspapers now, but once found untruthful stories hard to bear. Now he tries to be philosophical and believes truth will live and lies die. He says everybody in Terre Haute knows him, infirmities and all, and he is sure old and young, black and white, rich and poor, can say nothing against him.

"A man hasn't anything, after all, but his reputation," he observed, "and if he won't defend that it's because it isn't worth defending."

"Don't you think you could do labor some good by lecturing through the country?" I asked.

"There are two things I won't do," he replied promptly. "I won't write a book or lecture for money. I think it would be disreputable to thus take advantage of the notoriety I gained through workingmen's trouble. If I can survive all the talk, then I think I can do some good. If it's temporary notoriety then I shall, as a New York paper suggested, go into that obscurity from which I emerged.

"If I ever get time," Mr. Debs said, earnestly, "I want to devote some study to prisoners.

During the heat of the excitement over the last strike I was arrested and spent eight days in the Chicago jail. I would not give up that experience for any consideration. There were fifty women and five hundred men in that jail and it was marvelous to see the bond of comradeship that existed among them. All the time I was there I was deluged with food and flowers. I distributed them among the other prisoners, and if I gave a man a cigar, he would cut it in two or three and divide with friends. There was more fellowship among them than I have ever seen elsewhere in my life. Poor fellows! They are confined four to a small cell, and they are in that cell twenty-two out of the twenty-four hours. It is horrible.

"I became very friendly with all the men," he continued, "and I am willing to believe that if I had put them on their honor and let them out for so many hours every one of them would have returned at the appointed time.

"I had a funny letter from one of the prisoners after my conviction," Mr. Debs said, smiling. "He began it 'Dear Brother—I am glad to hear you got six months,' he wrote, 'and that you're coming back to us. You'll be welcomed with open arms.' "

Woman's Rights

In a little while I changed the subject by asking the convicted labor leader what he thought of woman's rights.

"Woman's suffrage is one of my hobbies," he said enthusiastically. "I believe in women having all the rights men have. Until they do, I do not think we are civilized. I firmly believe every social condition will be improved if women have the right to vote. Women have more integrity, more honor than men. A woman's vote couldn't be bought with a drink of whiskey. If I have done any good I owe it entirely to the influence of my mother, my wife and my sisters.

"Marriage is another hobby of mind," he added, earnestly. "I think it is brutal for a woman to take a husband merely for the sake of getting married or being supported. I think this alleged reproach for a woman staying single or being an old maid, is wrong. All honor to a woman, I say, who stays single because she does not find a congenial mate and is courageous enough to refuse anything else. I call it brave and deserving credit instead of reproach.

"My brother and I always declared our sisters should never marry unless they loved. Without any prompting from any one we secretly vowed that one of us would never marry while our sisters were single and by so doing, possibly force them to consider marrying for the sake of a home. And we didn't. My three sisters were married and the fourth engaged when I became engaged."

"Are you religious?" I asked. "I think I have heard you called an infidel."

"I don't subscribe to any creed," he replied gravely, "nor do I profess any religion. I am not an unbeliever. I accept the Christ standard as the highest

119

standard of morality, I believe in the religion of the golden rule. I wouldn't if I could disturb the religion of any human creature. Whatever a man's creed may be, if he sincerely believes it, it is the right creed. As for another world, I haven't time to think about it. I am interested in doing all the good I can in this."

"But don't you think it comforting to believe we'll meet those we love in another life?" I asked.

"It would be horrible not to think so," he answered, quickly. "I hate death; I never allow myself to think about it. It is enough to set one crazy. We've never had a death in our family. If I believed as Christians profess I would look on death as a benediction. I go to the extent of hoping, if I cannot believe, in an afterlife."

One of Mr. Debs' unbroken rules is not to receive presents or banquets. He says he does not think it right to let men give him what they can't afford to have for themselves, and that when he reads of managers and presidents of corporations receiving gifts as testimonials of esteem, he knows it is more a testimonial of slavery.

His Greatest Compliment

"The greatest compliment I ever had in my life was after we won a strike on the Great Northern for the section men. We got their wages raised from 80 cents a day to $1.25. The men wanted afterwards to give me a banquet, but I didn't think it right to look as if rejoicing over our victory. I would have no public demonstration. As my train drew out of the station the conductor asked me to come out on the platform, and there, lining either side of the railroad, were the section men, bent and worn from exposure, each man leaning on his shovel with his hat in his hand. It touched me deeply."

"Do you ever get blue."

"Sometimes; but I was never discouraged an instant in my life."

"How do you feel about the future for labor?" I asked.

"Very cheerful," he answered. "Government ownership of railroads is looming up in the distance. That will mean mutualism. I don't think we will ever have another great railroad strike, though there will be other strikes in other departments of industry.

"It would be foolish," he added, seriously, "to strike again. We know inevitably what the results will be. Courts will enjoin, authorities reprove them. With all the organized forces of society against them as well as the powers of government, failure is inevitable."

I asked Mr. Debs if I might stay and share his prison dinner, and he said he would be delighted to have me and wanted to have extra fare provided for me. I could scarcely make him understand that it was his fare I wanted to share.

Sheriff Eckert came in at 12.30 and Mr. Debs introduced me and explained my mission. The sheriff is a pleasant man and seems to think his prisoners are a well-behaved lot. We told him I wanted a photographer and he kindly offered to send for one.

It is a country jail and town and things are not conducted just as they might be in cities.

Three prisoners at a time are an event in Woodstock, so it is easy to understand the commotion raised by eight.

The only other thing that has ever happened in Woodstock was a hanging. A man killed an alderman in Chicago some years ago, and the man was taken to Woodstock and hanged. A pump now stands where the gallows stood, about fifteen feet from the jail window.

There are two prisoners in jail besides the labor leaders. One is a simple fellow, who could not get the wages due him from a niggardly old farmer, and so threatened to burn down his barn. The other is a German boy who stole silverware from his uncle.

At 1 o'clock Mrs. Eckert told us dinner was served and Mr. Debs and I went into the dining-room, where I was introduced to his seven comrades—William Burns, Sylvester Kellher, G. W. Howard, L. W. Rogers, R. M. Goodwin, James Hogan and M. J. Elliot.

The table was neatly spread and a bowl of soup stood at every plate. After the soup we had roast beef and boiled potatoes, Mr. Debs carving, and after that lemon pie for dessert. Everybody had a large cup of coffee.

The hour spent at dinner was most enjoyable. Everybody was in a good humor and everybody had a healthy appetite.

Then we went out into the sunlit corridor of the jail, where these men, if not admitted to bail, will spend most of their six months.

The corridor is long and narrow, with huge bars on one side and three large barred windows on the other. There were two tables strewn with books and papers, a shelf around the windows, also covered with books, and eight chairs, one of which was a barber's chair.

On the table was a small bunch of flowers, to which the men proudly called my attention.

Above the table was the picture of a bunch of violets.

The Prison Rules

Upon the wall were pinned the rules these men made and live up to. They rise at 6.30, have breakfast at 7.30. Breakfast consists of meat, potatoes, bread and coffee.

From 8 until 12 the men sit in the corridor in absolute silence, reading and studying. They have been active men, and stillness was a trial, so they impose a fine of 10 cents on every man who forgets and speaks aloud. This fine is given to the good, for, as Mr. Debs says, if wrong-doing be punished, it follows that goodness shall be rewarded.

So far four men have been fined, and Mr. Goodwin had the best record for goodness, so he won the reward—40 cents.

But that spoiled him and amid much laughter they told me that Mr. Goodwin had since then been fined twice!

Mr. Goodwin by the way is a relative of Nat Goodwin, the comedian, and the resemblance, except that Mr. Goodwin is more youthful, is very strong.

122

From 12 to 1 the men have what they call indifferently a "cake walk" and a "dress parade." At one they have dinner. At 2 o'clock they go into session again, and for the rest of the afternoon a pin could be heard drop.

From 6.30 until 7 they have supper, and afterwards they devote an hour to discussion, or as Mr. Debs says, "to good fellowship."

Someone proposes a subject, and they discuss it or what they have read during the day.

"We did tell stories at first." Mr. Debs said with his quick smile; "but we find after we've been in jail a week or so that we begin to repeat the same story four or five times. Then it isn't so funny."

At 9.30 sharp the solitary lamp, a hanging one, is put out, and everybody goes into his cell, and the good sheriff locks his prisoners up for the night.

The cells are small, with two cots to a cell, and two men are in each cell. There are only two tiers, comprising ten cells in all.

Each man makes his own bed. It is an iron cot fastened to the wall, and has a mattress, sheet, blanket and pillow.

Sometimes the men forget to make their beds, and then they are fined. One man had forgotten the day I was there, and he rushed into his cell hoping to escape notice until his work was done. But someone saw him, and amid great laughing he was pulled forth and made to pay his fine, which he did, blushing like a schoolboy.

The men have basins to wash in, three towels are provided the ten prisoners, and they have to last for two days.

Four men smoke and four do not. They may smoke when they wish.

I took a glance at their books. There was not a light work of fiction among them. The books were brought by the men from their homes.

"Intellectual Development of Europe," by Draper; "Social Problems," by Henry George; "Harvey's Coin Financial School," "Civilization Civilized," by Stephen Maybell; "Holy Bible," "Text-Book of Rhetoric,"

"Our Destiny," by Gronlund; "Better Days," by Fitch; "The Co-operative Commonwealth," by Gronlund, and volumes of Hawthorne and Shakespeare. That is only a small list, but it gives some idea of the style of reading enjoyed by these men who are fighting for workingmen's rights.

IN THE BIGGEST NEW YORK TENEMENT

Nellie Bly

The New York World/August 5, 1894

Nellie Bly Spends the Two Hottest Days of the Year in the largest "Double-Decker" in Town.

3,532 People in the Block

One Family Occupying Only Three Rooms Have Eight Boarders and Lodgers

Sleeping on the Fire-Escapes

No Scenes of Disturbance of Disorder Among the Throngs of Over-Crowded Tenants

Strange Phases of Life in a Big City

An Interesting Chat with the Janitress of the Big Double-Decker Tenement-House

The most thickly populated spot on earth?

That is where I've spent the two hottest days we've had this summer—last Saturday and Sunday.

Three thousand five hundred and thirty-two people in one block! Actually in one block, Second street on the south, Third street on the north, Avenue B on the west and Avenue C on the east.

No other block upon this earth, or same space of ground, is so densely populated. At least so it is claimed and, so far as statistics go, proved.

Thirty-five hundred and thirty-two people would make a good-sized town, and towns of smaller population have a mayor, a postmaster, constables, churches and bankers all of their own.

In one of the big tenements on this block, No. 228 Second street, an apartment was hired for me, and on Saturday afternoon, when everybody else was taking a half-holiday and thanking heaven they were able to be out of the hot city over Sunday, I moved into my new abode.

My first intention was to dress very poorly, so as to look as much as possible like those with whom I was to live, but on second consideration, I decided that I had never found any excuse for the dirty poor, and that if I was to be poor it was not necessary to be also ragged and dirty. So I wore a plain gray skirt, a shirt-waist and a sailor hat, and in a small hand-satchel carried all the toilet articles I needed.

Although I was partly prepared for the crowded appearance of the block, still at the first sight of it I thought something must have occurred to cause such numbers of people to congregate in one spot.

The sidewalks were well-nigh impassable, but making my way along slowly, I soon found my number and, climbing over the people upon the dirty stoop, stood upon the threshold of a new and strange existence.

Into the Tenement

The hall was dirty and dark and forbidding. It seemed well-filled with children. I addressed a half-grown girl and asked for the housekeeper.

The girl shook her uncombed head; she could not speak English. I spoke to another, a smaller girl with thin, stringy hair and one solitary sleeveless slip between her and nudeness. I inquired for the janitress.

"The housekeepers in there, if that's what you want," she answered, pointing to the first door in the hall.

The door was open. It opened into a very small kitchen. The kitchen opened into another room, a parlor, they call it, which was in front and was the only room that had direct light, it having a window facing the street. The kitchen also opened into a back room, a small, dark bedroom. There was a big stove in the middle of the kitchen and in the stove was a roaring fire, although the day was the hottest New York has been afflicted with in years.

I could not help glancing at the hot stove and from it to the small rooms on either side, and I wondered if some way could not be found to compel the builders of tenements to use some thought for the comfort of the unfortunate poor who must help to pay the 14 percent interest on the money invested. The kitchen build between the two living rooms may save money for the builders, but it means frightful discomfort for those who do not know what "a few weeks in the country" means.

'Are You Mrs. Brown?'

They must eat, and naturally to eat must cook, and a fire in the stock makes the other rooms, especially the rear bedroom, insufferably hot. Seeing me standing there the housekeeper left something she was looking after on the stove to come to me.

"An apartment was rented in this house for me, I believe," I said to her. And she looked at me with a smile. "I will take you up," she said, and she hurried into the rear room for the keys.

She led the way up the narrow, dirty stairs. I knew they were dirty, although I could see no more than I can at midnight when it is moonless and stormy; the vile stench made seeing superfluous.

With the instinct so exquisitely developed in dogs, I followed the housekeeper up the dark stairs, around a dark landing pregnant with the smothering smell of cabbage, and up a second flight. There she stopped and unlocked a door opening into a front apartment. They key was bent, and it took some time to accomplish this task; which being done, I walked into my new home.

Oh, the smell of it! It seemed to me that more than a million kinds of smell rushed out to embrace me in strong, if unseen, arms.

"Your furniture come, and I had 'em bring it here," she explained, pointing to a pile of stuff upon the floor. There it was, sure enough—furniture that had been bought for my use in the tenement.

127

In Nellie Bly's Room

I glanced at the floor; it was black with filth left by the last tenant, and a sickening smell seemed to run from it....

...'tain't safe to leave 'em open when you go out," the housekeeper explained. "There hasn't been anything taken yet, but it's better to be safe."

She opened the dust-covered windows as she spoke, and then she brought me one of my two new chairs.

"Will you scrub for me?" I asked, "and put things to place?"

She promised readily enough.

"I need odd jobs," she said.

Her arm was strong and willing, and in a short time the floor was as clean as it would come, and so hot was it that the wet boards dried almost as they were scrubbed. In fact, when she reached the doorside the entire floor was dry.

Then she set up the cot bed for me, put a chair at each of the front windows and a small table between them. My apartment consisted of three rooms, just like the housekeeper's; the front room, then the kitchen, in which there was running water, and the dark rear bedroom.

The rent was $10.50 a month and 75 cents deposit for the keys.

The rent is lower and the rooms are better than in the town of Pullman.

There was no way to have any cooking done in my apartment, so I went uptown for my dinner, returning to my new rooms about 9.30.

Everybody on the Street

Making my way through a task that looked impossible, I went to my room and opening my window, leaned out on the fire-escape to watch the strange scene below.

The pavement on both sides of the street was filled with a mass of human beings. A woman sitting on the curb pushed a carriage containing two babies arm's length and back. Another woman held a fretful child in her arms and kept balancing from one foot to the other to keep it quite. Four men clad in undershirts and trousers sat in chairs placed in a row on the curb. A woman was huddled down in a doorway, a shawl over her head and her face hidden between her knees. A group on a neighboring stoop were drinking turn about from a tin pail. An old man with an enormous beard and a long Dutch pipe stood smoking thoughtfully at the entrance to a dark hallway. A line of baby carriages, twelve in number, stood one after the other along the edge of the pavement, each carriage held one or two babies, and no one was in attendance.

Across the street, between the baker's and barber's front windows, was a soda fountain with three bottles of syrup, four long glasses and a mite of a showcase, a foot square, containing tobacco.

A bald-headed man sat hatless and coatless on a high stool behind the counter. Occasionally he sold a glass of soda to a woman or a child, or a package of cigarettes, with a picture and box of matches thrown in to a boy.

The strangest thing of all to me was the constant sound of voices which rose in one unbroken buzz from the street. Its like I never heard before, and so strange was it that I can find no words to describe it. It was one loud, continuous sound, much, I fancy, as would come from a mob advancing upon something. It was a distinct but distant sound, a constant buzz, with no distinguishable words. Within the tenement where I lived everything was comparatively still. It seemed to me that everybody must be out in the street.

After a while the housekeeper came to see me. She brought me a glass and pitcher and said she could buy the ice across the street.

She Was a "Widow," Too

She returned with the ice. She put it in a pitcher and ran water over it. The water was thick with a black sediment, which finally settled in the bottom of the pitcher. She placed the pitcher and a glass upon the mantel for my service. I noticed that she looked lonely, so I asked her to sit down.

"Are you all alone?" she asked me bluntly.

I had to account for the "Mrs.," which the man upon whom had fallen the duty of renting the room had credited to me, so I told her I was a widow.

"I'd never thought you were married, you look that young," she said, and then she signed.

"Are you a widow also?" I asked, for it seemed she wanted me to ask.

"Yes," she replied. "But my husband ain't dead yet," she added with an afterthought.

I looked at her curiously.

"He can't live with me," she explained. "He's on Ward's Island; gone in his head, you know."

"Ah! That is sad," I say, sympathetically, and I see her dark eyes fill with tears.

Her eyes have the sad, appealing look of a dog, and I remember that is her hair is tossed and untidy, her little rooms are spotlessly clean, and I like her.

"He was a good man," she says, encouraged by my sympathy, "but he couldn't sleep nights. That's what was wrong with him. He never slept nights and his head ached so all the time. But he was such a good man."

"Could nothing be done to make him sleep?" I asked.

Husband on Ward's Island

No; he was always taking everything, everything he read about or people told him about, but it didn't help, so the doctors said I'd better send him to Ward's Island. They said he'd get worse all the time, and when he couldn't work I couldn't keep him because they said it wasn't safe to leave him alone, so he had to go to the Island."

"Do you ever see him?"

"I go to see him every two weeks. I was there today, but he seemed bright today. 'Why do you keep me here?' he said to men, an' he cried. 'Wasn't I always a good man to you? Won't you take me home?'

"That's what makes it hard," she said with quivering lips. "He was a good man to me always and to the children. So kind and quiet! He never said a cross word, even when his poor head ached so."

"Is there no hope for his recovery?" I asked.

"No; the doctors say he has—I don't know what you call it; his brain is all soft. He'll get worse all the time, but they say he can live to be an old man; outlive me, for he won't be working and I will. I never had to work hard when he was with me. He was such a good man! That's what makes it hard."

She told me she had five children, the youngest about two and the eldest about ten.

"I worked hard, took in washing and went out cleaning and everything, but I couldn't get enough to keep them, so I had to give the three oldest ones to the home. They'll be kept there till they're sixteen an' I can see them once a month."

Making Both Ends Meet

"It's better for them," she added, as if to assure me of her rightful intentions. "It keeps them off the street, an' my man wouldn't have liked them to grow up in the streets, an' they'll get a schooling."

"Yes; I should think they are much better off. How do you keep yourself now, and your two little ones?"

"I get my rent free for taking care of this house," she replied. "That's a good saving. Then I do washings or any work I can get. Work has been scarce for a year now, but I've had two boarders; two young ladies. They work in a cloak factory and they make $5 a week. I charge them $2.50 each for their board and wash. But they are going to leave Monday. The one is getting married and the other is going with her. I don't know what I'll do then."

131

A child came running upstairs for the housekeeper.

"The new people are down there," the child said, and the housekeeper said she must go.

"It's a newly married couple that's movin' in tonight," she explained.

"Rather a large move, isn't it?" I asked.

"Yes; but he wanted to help with it after his work," she said. "I left the lights burning in the hall because they were coming. I always put them out at 10."

Midnight, and I sat at my window watching the crowd below.

Midnight Noises and Sights

The boys on the trucks made attempts to sing; children still darted hither and thither; men and women clustered on the sidewalks; that strange buzz of life was just as loud as ever.

Will they never go to bed? I wondered.

The noise, that unearthly buzz, exhausted me. I felt that I needed sleep and that I would be unable to get any. The bad odors from the street and house had made my head ache.

Then lights came in a few of the windows opposite and men and women and children, each in a single undergarment, moved around as if making ready for bed. There was no attempt to close the shutters or left down the blinds.

I lay down upon my cot and tried to sleep. People came up and went downstairs, stumbling in the dark or striking matches against the wall to give them light. The newly wedded couple below me were hammering their furniture together. The baby in the apartment overhead was crying lustily.

I may have slept five minutes; it couldn't have been longer. The baby overhead screamed so lustily and angrily that I felt half inclined to go up

132

to see what was wrong with it. Somewhere else in the house I could hear a baby-carriage being wheeled back and forth on the bare floor to keep some child quiet.

I got a book and read.

The Fire-Escape for Beds

At 2 o'clock I went to my window. The bald-headed, hatless and coatless man at the soda-fountain was just selling a strawberry soda to a little girl who had to get on her tiptoes to reach the top of the counter. The men and boys were no longer attempting to sing, but were lying a dark mass in the bottom of the wagons. The line of baby carriages had disappeared. One woman on the pavement beneath my window sat upright on a chair and kept a baby-carriage in constant motion with her foot.

I noticed a little dark heap of something on the fire-escape near my window. I could have put out my hand and touched it, but I didn't.

I merely watched it. Presently above the bundle of rags I saw a little curly head toss restlessly. A little girl was sleeping there.

I leaned out of the window and looked about. Beneath my fire-escape lay a man in his underclothes; a little beyond him slept a woman and child.

Because of the intervening bedclothing I could not see those upon the fire-escapes above, but I could get a view of the other side of the block and every fire-escape was transformed into a bed. The buzzing in the street never ceased; fewer people were moving about, though just as many as ever were sitting around as if they meant to spend the night where they were.

It was now nearly 3 o'clock in the morning. I went back to my cot so sleepy that I felt I should no longer mind the frightful heat, the smell and noise. Notwithstanding my weariness I laughed to find that the reporter who had been sent to buy my necessary household articles had only bought me one bedcover. It was a heavy woolen blanket!

And it was the hottest night in six years! And what was infinitely worse, to protect myself from mosquitoes I had to cover up!

I was so miserable and uncomfortable that I went to sleep, and when I woke again two babies, in place of one, were scratching matches against my door.

I went to the window and found little change in the street below. The woman still sat stiffly upright in a chair, rolling her baby carriage with her foot, and the bald man at the soda fountain was sitting upon his high stool with folded arms and motionless.

Then a milk wagon rattled up to a shop opposite, and the driver deftly tossed five filled cans on the pavement and five empty cans into his wagon. Then he yelled to the storekeeper and rattled the garden door; the other wasn't closed.

…Sneider by this time was holding the screen door open the milkman whirled the cans inside. The quickness with which Sneider made his appearance proved that he had not undressed to go to bed. Nor did he return for a second snooze. He opened up shop at once, and as customers had not appeared, came out and sat before his open door.

I went to my cot again. When I woke the babies were still crying upstairs and the mosquitoes had disappeared, but their places were taken by busy, buzzing flies. I looked out upon the street. The soda-fountain man was still motionless on his high stool and the woman still sat by her baby carriage. A new woman had appeared. She was pacing up and down the pavement for the matter of ten feet, with a child in her arms. The child's face in the early daylight wore the color of death.

The people still slept on the fire-escapes, but the men had disappeared from the wagons, curbs and door-stoops.

The heat and the constant noise had worn me out. The air in my room was stifling and had a heavy, vile smell. Still, I went to sleep and slept on until 8 o'clock.

Only One Sunday Paper

I went out for breakfast and came back to my post of duty a few hours later.

134

I found the strange block once again jammed with people. All the little shops, the butcher, the baker, the coal dealer and ice-man, the candy shops and the soda fountain, were wide open, doing business just as if it were a week day.

I noticed that in the entire block only one man had a Sunday newspaper. No one else read.

I also noticed that families had no particular hour for meals and that there was no ceremony about eating together. I also noticed that they mostly ate something with a spoon out of a bowl.

Just opposite three children were sleeping on a fire-escape, and above them two men in their under-clothing and bare feet took turns at drinking out of a broken pitcher, and on the fire-escape, still above them, a little boy of bilious yellow, clad only in a short shirt, kept crying to some boys in the street below, and never getting a reply: "Do you want a pussy-cat? Do you want a pussy-cat?"

As the day advanced the line of baby-carriages made its appearance upon the pavement, increasing steadily with the shade. The soda-water man did a pretty good business and the ice-man had constant customers. In fact, all the shop-keepers, including the barber, who, like the other men, wore only his undershirt and trousers, did a good-steady business.

I saw no fights and no disorder all the time I was there and I saw a policeman upon the block only once. The nearest approach to trouble was with an amateur baseball team who were howling themselves hoarse and bumping into everything in their limited field in the street.

At last the ball hit a small occupant of a carriage in the baby-carriage line, and a big, fat, dirty man with a pipe in his mouth yelled lustily for the baker's wife, and the baby squalled like a young Indian. The baker's wife ran out, wrapping up some cakes as she ran, and the baker, with his hands and arms covered with flour, came up out of the basement. Everybody clustered around the baby and the barker barber walked off in triumph with the ball, shaking his fist at the boys when they yelled "Hi, there!" to throw it back.

A Little Boy Visitor

A timid knock came upon my door, and I opened it to find there a pretty little boy in a white waist, and with his hair just as nicely brushed as it could be. He had big, trusting blue eyes, and he looked up at me and smiled, saying, pityingly, "Ain't you lonesome?"

I told him I was, a little bit, because I didn't want him to think I didn't want to see him, and I asked him in and gave him a chair at the window.

His mother, who proved to be my neighbor in the rear, followed him in to explain that the child knew I was alone and thought he would come in to cheer me up.

Then I talked with the mother. She told me the house was the kind known as a "double-decker tenement," and that there were four apartments to a floor, two front and two rear, of three rooms each.

She also told me that the largest family in the house numbered eleven, all of whom lived in three small rooms. She said that nearly all the people in the house kept boarders, and that there were three empty apartments at present and fewer people in the house than usual.

117 Persons Under One Roof

We counted the number of persons under the one roof.

There were, by actual count, one hundred and seventeen people!

The largest family numbered eleven. The smallest was my own.

The family that lived above me have twins. It was the twins that cried all night—sometimes solos, sometimes duets. The woman who sat on the pavement all night did so because her child is very ill and the night air is better for it than that of the hot, stifling rooms.

Her son and my little visitor had been at death's door with diphtheria four weeks ago. For eight days and nights she sat without sleep or rest by his bedside, and then the doctor who told her to prepare for the worst at 10.30

one night shook hands with her at 6 and told her the little chap had "pulled through."

She hadn't cried before, but she cried then and cried herself to sleep. Her husband couldn't sit up at night, because he had to work to provide food for them. The husband is a clerk in a hat store and gets $10 a week. He works from 7.30 until 10.30 every day, Sundays as well as week days.

Since her boy got well, four weeks ago, two other children had died in the house, and a man, the father of the eleven children. He died very suddenly of inflammation of the brain. Thirteen of them lived in the three small rooms.

When he was dying, she told me, the eleven children and the wife gathered around the bed and cried so loud and went on so that he couldn't die; they wouldn't let him. He was dead, she declared, but their wild lamentations made him come back to life.

Then a friend came in and said: "You must go away; he can't die if you don't." And though it was because he was dying they cried so, yet they went out and gave him the chance. I thought if I had been one of the eleven and crying would have kept my father alive, nothing would have induced me to stop, but I didn't tell her my thoughts.

They weren't gone five minutes, she added, until the poor man closed his eyes, sighed gently and was dead. He could die when they didn't cry.

IN TRINITY'S TENEMENTS

Nellie Bly

The New York World/December 17, 1894

Nellie Bly Visits Many Miserable Homes Owned by That Corporation

Wretchedness and Squalor

Outrageous Rents for Filthy Dens in Foul, Rickety, Leaky, Unsanitary Hovels

Death, Too, Lurks in Many of Them

You Will Learn Here Something About the Real Life of Dismal New York

Trinity! Meaning the Father, the Son and the Holy Ghost. Embracing everything that means love, mercy, justice, charity.

The Trinity corporation is rich beyond the dreams of avarice. It was within its power to solve the tenement-house question, to use its vast wealth to benefit the poor, but what has it done?

I will tell you.

They have been spending thousands of dollars to celebrate Christmas, ordering masses of green foliage and holly and mistletoe to delight the eye, and a special musical programme to charm the ear, while I have been visiting their poor tenants in their miserable tenements.

I happened by chance to go first to No. 4 Grand street. I did not know the part of the city in which the Trinity property is mainly located, and when the Grand street car suddenly swung around a corner and the conductor

138

pointed down a street that stopped abruptly and went nowhere, as the end, or rather the beginning, of Grand street, I was somewhat surprised.

I alighted and walked down the block, looking closely at the houses. They were small red brick houses, presenting rather a respectable appearance for a poor locality. Near the end of the street I saw a small dilapidated frame two-story and attic.

THE FIRST GLIMPSE OF SQUALOR

An empty wagon stood in the street and an ash can, overflowing and vile-smelling, was on the shaky frame stoop. There was no number upon the house, and though some inner instinct told me it was the one for which I searched, still I could scarcely believe it. But on looking closer I saw a badly made figure 4 in chalk upon the dirty door.

There was no knob with which to fasten the door, so I entered and found myself in a dark, dirty and ill-smelling hall. The floor was not carpeted, but it certainly was not bare. A layer of filth, the accumulation doubtless of months, covered it.

A knock upon the two doors leading to the rooms on the first floor was not answered, so I went up a flight of rickety stairs, four one way, then a sharp turn and three the other, and I was on a landing from which opened two doors.

I knocked upon the one nearest. It was opened by a little, clean-faced old woman, bent in form and sad of countenance. I told her briefly that I was looking at the Trinity tenements, and with her permission, would like to see her rooms.

The door was opened wide and I was invited to enter. I am used to tenements and sights of poverty, but the picture of misery that confronted me stirred me deeply.

The room was small, about one and a half times the width of a single bed, and one and a quarter times the length. A single bed that crossed two windows just managed to leave space enough for the door to open. At the end of the room and the foot of the bed was a small cook stove. Two wooden chairs, one with the bottom split and the other without a back, and a rickety table completed the furniture. A few ragged clothes hung upon

139

the door, a wooden bucket containing water sat on the floor, and one cup, one plate, a dish and two knives were on the table.

That was all the room contained except three unhappy people—the little old woman, her daughter and her son-in-law, who lay upon the dirty bed propped up against the headboard, for pillow he had none. His face was thin and pale, and his breathing was loud and laborious.

"Are you ill?" I asked rather foolishly, for my eyes had answered my question.

"Yes," he replied slowly, and in a husky voice, "I had two hemorrhages Monday, and I'm feeling pretty bad."

I asked him questions, and he told me his story modestly and without complaint. He is a glass packer, but has been out of work for many months, except such odd jobs as he could obtain. Once he carried sample cases for a Maiden lane jewelry drummer. It was during the very cold and wet weather we had a few weeks since. The cases weighed 106 pounds and he carried them, drenched to the skin and shivering with the cold, to Harlem.

ONE TENANT'S MISERY

That brought on his first sickness. Two weeks ago he got work at No. 72 Murray street at his trade. On Monday, as he left work he had the hemorrhages, and doubtless by the time he is able to go back to work the work will be over for the season, as it is ended when Trinity rings in the New Year.

Still, the man must have shelter while he lives. And although the rain comes in the windows, which are pasted over with paper to do the service of glass, his room is infinitely better than the streets. Cook, eat and sleep in it, for the outrageous price of $2 a week.

There are eight apartments (so called) in the building. One in the basement, consisting of two rooms, for which the charge is $5 a week. The basement is dark, filthy and damp. On the first floor the price for the front room is $2.50 a week and $3 for the rear room. The prices are the same on the second floor, and the hall room is $1.25. In the attic are two pens called rooms for which the tenants pay $6 a month.

The only water is in the yard, a small space, filthy, ill-smelling and filled with pools of stagnant water. The closet, one for the entire house, has no roof and its floor is unsafe. It stands within a foot of the hydrant.

The tenants of the first floor and the basement were out, but on the floor where I found the sick man I saw in the front room an old woman partially paralyzed.

The plaster in the corner of her room was wet where the rain comes through the side of the house. In some places the plastering had fallen down and in all places it was filthy dirty. The floor was warped and uneven.

This old woman is supported by her daughter, a ragpicker who works from 7 A.M. until 6 P.M. for $4 a week, and then, owing to the dull times, is laid off more than half the week.

The hall-room tenant was out, so I felt my way up a twisting and dark stair, so narrow that two persons could not pass on it, and so twisted that I felt every moment as if I would tumble down.

First at the head of five or more steps was a door, a few boards roughly pounded together and put on hinges. It had no knob. No door in the house had. The sick man's had a nail fastened to a string. Stumbling on a few steps with my head bumping against the rafters, I hit against another door which flies open at my touch and shows me a low and narrow passage with a window at the end, from which a woman is hanging clothes on a line.

She was a nice little French woman, very tidy. Her room, if I can call it such, was merely a little space under the roof.

At one side, where the roof ran up to the rafter, the height was probably five feet. At the other side, where it sloped down, one couldn't have found space between the roof and the floor to tack carpets. It was practically a case of making two ends meet—the roof and the floor of a house.

A QUAINT ATTIC PICTURE

There was one window in the place. It was the kind that is cut in the roof and built to stand out. To reach it one would have had to crawl across the single bed, which took all the space, except what was occupied by the wee cook-stove.

It was the smallest place I ever saw for two human beings to live in. But the little French woman had it as clean as a combination of soap, water and hard work can make it, and it wasn't her fault that the sickly geranium on the window-sill found it always too warm or too cold for health.

As I did not believe in judging the Trinity Corporation by their houses in one street, I decided to make a jump and see if I could not find better ones.

I went to Clarke street and I saw some good buildings that I thought were Trinity property, but when I inquired, I found that Trinity owned the ground, but lease-holders owned the buildings. I was told if I would go further up the street I would find four houses rented by Trinity. They were Nos. 9, 21-1/2, 26 and 28, the oldest, most dilapidated and disgraceful looking houses in the street.

No. 9 is a frame tenement of three stories. It is ready to fall down. The first floor is occupied by a toy and candy shop and is only one room deep. The proprietor lives on the floor above his shop and rents out the top floor for $6 a month. The water is in the back yard, a wet, dirty place, into which the sun never comes. There used to be a frame tenement in the rear, but the Health Board made the Trinity Corporation pull it down.

The floor in the house is anything but on the dead level, and even a short person could without the slightest difficulty touch the ceiling. For this the toy man pays $25 a month, and he thinks it's not very high, although he has to keep eightg black and white cats and one Skye terrier to keep the rats from carrying away his stock.

I went next to No. 28 Clarke street. It is an old frame that bears its misery on its face.

In the basement, where the floor looks like the deck of a ship in a heavy sea, I found a nice old Italian cobbler, with his wife and two children. The old couple could not speak English, but their little boy, with the ideal face of a poet, answered all my questions promptly, intelligently and politely.

THEY HELP SWELL THE FUND

His father sometimes didn't earn a dollar in a whole month, he said, but he had two other brothers, one a little bigger than him, who "made ties" in South fifth avenue. The biggest brother had had no work for a long time, but the other brother got $2 a week for stamping the name on "the ties." His sister worked on "coats," for which she got $3 a week.

The combined income, $5, had to keep them and pay their rent, $10 a month. Their rooms are three-quarters under the ground and flat upon it.

There is the front and back room, and between is a dark space divided by the passage which connects the two rooms. This dark space holds on either side two beds, which touch the wall at the head and at the foot.

The floor is warped and the walls are damp, but still trinity charges $10 a month for the place.

On the first floor of the house is the same arrangement of rooms, except that the width of the dirty hall is taken from them.

For this front and back room with the dark space between that will and does hold two beds, the family pays $14 a month. The floor in these rooms is worn out, has been many years, but Trinity will not repair it and the family have been compelled to do so themselves.

"The Trinity carpenter said that the Trinity Corporation was like a woman," observed the girl I found in these rooms. "If she found a small hold she would patch it, but when it gets to be a big one she things it's useless to do anything and so she lets it go."

Of course there are many places uptown where for $14 a month this family could hire a four or six room flat, where they would have a bath, range and running water. But they cannot live uptown. Their work is downtown, and they must be near it. The two sons drive trucks when they have work, and the daughter works at feathers, and they together keep the father and mother.

By going up dirty and uncertain stairs, stairs that aren't mates, or even any relation to each other, I found on the second floor an Italian family that had lived there for twenty-six years. Their rooms corresponded with those

143

below which I have already described. There are no accommodations whatever, unless running water in the hall is considered by Trinity a modern improvement. For these four rooms the family pays $12.50, and the rent has never been reduced in the twenty-six years, although the house has been growing older and poorer all the while.

And never until this month has the family been compelled to ask the wealthy Trinity Corporation to wait for its rent, the woman told me proudly, and she added that they had been very nice about.

Considering that they have paid in rent the entire price of the house, lacking only $6.50, one would suppose the agent might be "nice" about waiting a day or two.

And that is the only thing I found in all my investigation that was "nice" about the Trinity Corporation.

A CRIB UNDER THE EAVES

On the top floor, if you could ever summon up enough courage to feel your way through blinding darkness to it, you will find a landing with four doors facing each other in space literally not large enough to turn around in.

The one door is from the stairs; the others open into "apartments." Had I not been told that people lived there I should certainly never have suspected it and never have found them.

As it was I pounded upon the wood I felt in the darkness and a man opened a door and reluctantly admitted me to his home.

I have heard of birds that build their nests under the eaves of houses, but I never knew human beings to have homes there until I visited Trinity's tenements.

This man's room was like the one I saw at No. 4 Grand street, only worse. It was smaller and poorer.

A bed stood under the slanting roof at one side; a crib shared the other side with a small stove. Between them was the space of about two feet. It was occupied by a cradle, rather cleverly made of a soap-box, pivoted at either

144

end to two upright pieces of wood. It was certainly not a swinging brass bed, as one sees in the shop windows, but it was built in that style.

The man and I stood at the door. Of course, it was practically impossible to enter the room, or whatever one may call it. We could stand where we were because that happened to be the highest place in the roof, but even a wee baby mouse couldn't crawl where the roof met the floor.

Still that man, his wife and three children eat, sleep and live in that place. He has not been able to work for many months because he has heart disease, but he can mind the children while his wife goes out to get what work she can—washing, scrubbing, anything—to help make up $4,50 a month so the wealthy and charitable Trinity corporation will permit them to go on living under the eaves.

Trinity has three other "apartments" on this "floor." They are all like the one I saw, so the man said. One is occupied by an old man and woman, who go out to work every day, and the other is occupied by an old man, who works all day, but, so far as is known, is absolutely alone in the world.

They pay $4.50 for each apartment, which means $13.50 for the floor; $12.50 for the floor below, $14 for the first floor and $10 for the basement, makes in all $50 a month for the miserable old tenement, which is estimated by Trinity as being worth $4,500.

Pretty comfortable interest on their money.

After that I visited a number of Trinity houses. At first I went to some that looked respectable and comfortable, thinking to be able to write that all was not black, but that the wealthy corporation had good as well as miserable buildings for their tenants.

But I was sadly disappointed. Although I spent three days looking after their dwellings in a totally unbiased and conscientious manner, I must state with regret that I soon learned one unmistakable fact:

If a house was painted and had a comfortable look from the outside, it was a Trinity leasehold, and its appearance was totally due to the owner.

145

On the other hand, if the house was the most dilapidated and disreputable-looking in the entire block, it was owned and rented solely by the Trinity corporation.

Nor did I visit houses in one street alone and base my judgment on them, but made my tour as varied as possible among the houses owned by Trinity in Greenwich Village.

At No. 82 Vandam street I found a miserable two-story and attic frame building, with a collection of poor but interesting tenants.

Going down several steps into a basement that is almost entirely below the street, I found a neat housewife, as I judged by the tidy curtains at the windows.

She had only two rooms, the front one being a kitchen, dining-room and bedroom, and a rear cellar room, the air of which gave me a chill, serving as second bedroom and containing two beds, which left a space scarcely a foot in width between them.

The poor rooms were as neat as hard work could make them, and the woman was herself as clean as a new pin.

She was such a nice, motherly old lady; the kind that wins one's heart by a simple glance at her sweet face and white hair, and mild eyes that look straight at one and whose frankness shows that in their whole life they had never one wicked thought or deed to conceal.

I found her in the back yard, vainly trying to pile some good earth around the roots of a tree that had managed to live a starved existence in that poor locality. I love trees as much as I love all dumb animals, and so I naturally felt my heart go out to the dear old English woman.

"Certainly, miss, you may see my rooms," she said in reply to my inquiry, never asking my object.

And when I had seen them, and she told me the rent–$5.50 a month—and I had involuntarily said something about the outrageous price, she said quietly:

ENGLISH RENTS CHEAPER

"Do you think that much, miss? I have been told that was low rent for America. We have lived here three years, ever since we came over, and I had no way to know what rent was just."

"How does your rent compare with your rent in England," I asked anxiously.

"Well, miss," she answered, with a smile, "it is vastly different. I only know about Liverpool, where we always lived. We had a nice house there with six rooms; a better house in all, miss, than this, and with it we had a nice garden. For it we paid six six a week, for, you know, miss, we pay our rent by the week there instead of by the month as we do here."

I asked her how much "six six" was in our money, and she said she thought it was about $1.00.

In this family are the husband and wife, one boy, who "follows the sea," it being also the father's trade; two girls and an orphaned niece about fourteen years old. The husband has been unable to work for fifteen weeks owing to a sore leg. One girl lives out, but has no place at present, and the other earns $3.50 a week in a biscuit factory.

There is one other member of the family, a very dear one. It is a green parrot with a black bill and yellow spot at the back of his neck. He calls the nice old lady "Mamma!", whistles beautifully and sings with a decided cockney accent "After the Ball is Over."

The floor above this interesting family is divided into two apartments, consisting of two small rooms each. The front rents for $8 a month and the back for $5.50. I did not see either, as the families were out.

From the yard one can walk up a flight of some ten or fifteen stairs to the second floor. It is also divided into two apartments. The front rooms are occupied by a woman whose husband goes to sea. She never speaks to any of the neighbors and has never been known to open her door in reply to any knock. However, all the neighbors know that she pays $7 a month for her rooms.

147

A little woman with a small baby in her arms admitted me to the rear rooms. The first room is small, and plumes on the hat of a medium sized woman would touch the ceiling.

The room was comfortably furnished, for the family once lived amid better surroundings.

The husband was a longshoreman, or, rather, the employer of longshoremen, a sober, industrious and saving workman. His wife was a neat and saving housekeeper, but exposure to all kinds of weather did its work, and five years ago the husband began to lose his strength.

He held out as long as he could, but the sickness was stronger than he, and now for ten months he has been unable to move from his bed, a victim of consumption.

DYING IN MISERY

There he lay, a mass of bones covered with a yellow skin. His soul seemed already to have gone beyond, for his eyes were dull and unseeing, giving me the same look of utter unconsciousness that he cast upon his wife and child.

"I have five children," the woman told me. "The eldest, a girl not yet sixteen, works in a laundry, for which she gets $4 a week. The boy next to her in age is an errand boy and is paid $3 a week. The boy next is at school and the one still younger you see out there in the yard cutting wood for me. The baby (the one in her arms) is not yet ten months old."

The family lives upon the $7 weekly income and pays $7 a month for their miserable rooms.

I was awfully glad there were three boys. They have to sleep in that bed on the boarded balcony. It must be dreadfully cold, and if it wasn't that there are three boys and that they have to sleep in a single bed, they would never be able to keep warm. And I am positive Trinity would not give them burial room if they froze to death.

They have to crawl over the foot of the bed to get in. I wonder if they ever laugh, and if they rush to see who'll get in first, and if they ever tumble each other over the footboard!

148

Or I wonder if the poor little errand boy is too tired to laugh and play, and if the mother makes the other boys keep still so he can rest, that he may be able to work like a grown man and bring home his poor little $3 every Saturday to help pay the rent to Trinity!

I went up the stairs to the attic. There I found a young widow with two small children. She proved to be one of my human birds, whose nest is under the eaves.

LEAKS! ALWAYS LEAKS!

The roof is high at one side and meets the floor at the other. It has never been boarded over, and the rafters are all black and the light of day shows through the crevices. A stove is fastened to a chimney that goes zig-zag, so that, while it starts near the side of the house, it comes out of the roof at the middle.

When it rains the water comes through on the floor, but the widow smiles as she says it can't hurt her carpet. She has some bits of worn oil-cloth, but water doesn't hurt them.

Sometimes the rain drowns out her kitchen fire and that makes her sorry, and when I showed her how wet and damp her walls were she said I must remember that the house must be very old!

She has to go to the yard for the water, as must every other tenant in the house. At night the halls are dark, but in the daytime any one would note how wonderfully clean and tidy the tenants keep them.

For this attic the widow pays Trinity $5.50. She does not complain, nor do any of the others.

I do say, in all my experience among tenements, I never found poorer tenements or better tenants. They are all extremely poor, but they are respectable, clean, and not of the whining, begging class.

An inexperienced person is apt to visit tenements and consider people poor according to their filth. Where they find clean rooms and people they are most likely to fail to note the poverty.

149

Among the poor in New York I never found as clean and respectable a class as I did in Greenwich village, though Trinity deserves no credit for that.

I next went to No., 88 Charlton street, and I never found a New York tenement so poor. It is a miserable old frame that has stood so many years that it's too tired to hold up much longer.

On the ground floor is a tailor shop, where a lot of men and women, who pretended not to understand English, sat sewing.

Through the low hall, from which the damp and dirty plastering is hanging, I went up the creaky and unsafe stairs to the landing on the second floor, where I knocked in the darkness until a ragged woman opened a door and let me enter.

She was a poor, miserable, unhappy-looking creature, and was vainly endeavoring to clean a place that can never be made clean.

I never saw walls and ceilings in such a state of filth and dilapidation.

She had this room and one inside that was perfectly dark and had the damp smell of a cellar. The woman made a light and showed me the floor and walls, but the smell was so intense that I asked her a few hurried questions and went away.

A MISERABLE PEN, THIS

Her husband is at sea, and she has been compelled to put her two boys in a Catholic home. Her girl, not yet sixteen years old, earns $4 a week in the Empire laundry, and on that they live, unless she happens to get a day's scrubbing.

She pointed to a hole in the ceiling where the plastering had fallen down, and she told me that she paid $8 a month for the miserable pen.

"I think it's a little too much rent," she said, timidly, "I don't think it's worth more than seven. The halls are dark and filthy, and you should see the yard! We have to carry out water up from it, and it's awful. I do think the rent's too much. It's all poor people can do to pay it."

I asked her what she knew about the Trinity Corporation—what it meant.

"They're landlords, that's all I know," she answered, which amused me very much.

Next door I found a man and two small and very dirty children in two rooms that beggar description. The filthy and falling walls, the uneven and broken floor, and glassless windows, I leave to the merciful imagination of my readers, who, if curiosity is strong enough, can visit the place.

When I spoke to the tall, dirty man he set the baby he held in his arms down on the floor, and pointing to his mouth, made signs that he was dump. I wrote on a bit of paper that I was looking at Trinity's tenements, and asked him how much rent he paid. He wrote in reply: "Eight dollars a month."

I shrugged my shoulders in disgust, and he held up his hands pitifully and helplessly.

I then wrote the following questions, to which he wrote the replies.

"How many children have you?"

"Three."

"Can you work at anything?"

"I am a longshoreman. No work."

"Does your wife work?"

"She is out peddling lace."

RICKETTY AND FOUL-SMELLING

Just them a pretty little girl not more than five years old came in with a loaf of bread under her arms. She said the man was her father, that her mother talked to him with her fingers, but she couldn't say much to him. She tried, moving her lips and her little thin arms, but he failed to understand her.

151

At No. 35 Watts street I found the front house is rented by a respectable widow, who pays Trinity $40 for it and sublets to tenants.

I also learned by this time that many of the Trinity houses are like the corporation—they present a good front.

Many of their old houses have a brick front, which, being painted, is apt to make a casual observer consider the houses very comfortable ut a glance at the miserable frame rears dispelled this delusion.

The rear of No. 35 Watts street is worse even than the yard house back of it, though that is bad enough, It is the only yard house the Fire Commissioners left standing. A short time ago every one of Trinity's houses had houses in the rear.

In this rear house are two apartments on one side, consisting of two wee cubby-holes, for which the family on the first floor pay $6 a month and the one on the second floor pay $9.

On the next side the apartment on the first floor consists of one room, for which $5 is paid, and on the second and top floor is a room the shape of a flatiron, and scarcely larger, with a small adjoining closet that Trinity calls "room," for which $5 is paid also.

MISERY PAYS THE TOLL

The walls and plastering are in a frightful condition. The water is in the yard.

The front and rear houses are estimated at $6,000. The rent collected by Trinity for the same is $85 per month.

No. 259 Houston street is estimated at $5,000 value. It is one of a long row of Trinity houses, but all the others are leased to tenants who sublet. No. 259 has always been leased, too, but the policeman who had it last said he could not make it pay and gave it up.

Two nice old women with snow-white hair live in the basement. They have been tenants of Trinity for the last thirty years. They keep their two basement rooms spotlessly clean and tidy, and it is entirely due to them that the paper on the wall is new and clean and that the ceiling, just an inch or so above our heads, is whitewashed.

But they cannot prevent the floor from being on the slide, nor can they stop the green mould from coming on the damp walls in the hallo, or the green moss from covering the stones in the areaway.

When it rains the water forms in deep pools in the areaway and they have to dip it out, but still Trinity charges them $5 a month for living there.

The first floor has a front and a back room, with two dark rooms between, for which Trinity receives $15 a month. Eighteen dollars a month they get for the second, and the top is divided into two apartments, consisting of two rooms each, for which Trinity receives $9 from each family.

The widow in the rear top rooms is to be dispossessed. She has a boy who used to earn something by "putting in" coal, but he's been in the hospital for weeks now with spinal trouble. She has two girls. One scarcely twelve was a nurse in some family, but she is homesick. The other girl, a tall, thin, underfed soul, who was frying some foul-smelling fish, said she worked in a candy factory for four years. She used to earn as much as $4.50 a week, but work got slack and slacker, and now she has none at all.

That makes $60 a month Trinity receives on a $5,000 house. The majority of the other homes in the block are leased yearly for $66 a month.

I called at scores of other houses, but as the story of them is the same as that already told of others, I shall not enter into a description of each one. In the rear of No. 12 Clarkson street I found some interesting people. I first looked at the dirty yard and cellar, there being pools of water standing in each.

Then I went in to see the tenement. It and the adjoining one, No. 10, have four floors, with two families to a floor. The halls are narrow, dirty and dark, and the apartments consist of one front room and one small pen dignified by the name of bedroom. Both houses are as filthy and damp as can be imagined, and there is much sickness among the tenants.

The same scale of outrageous prices are charged. For the ground floor $10, $5 for each apartment; $11, or $5.50 each for the second and third floors, and $9, or $4.50 each, for the top floor.

153

THE CEILING IS FALLING

On the second floor I found a woman who has lived there for seventeen years next June. Eight years ago her husband died and left her four children to provide for.

She succeeded beautifully. There is no water in the house, but every day of her life this energetic woman carried enough water up from the yard to do a washing. The clothes she had to dry in the one room in which they lived, as the bed fills the other.

Now she does not labor so hard, for one girl lives out, another is a "saleslady" (the mother tells me with pride) and the boy is in a grocery, leaving the little girl at home with her good mother.

In all these seventeen years Trinity has never done any repairing for their worthy widow tenant. Once she papered the rooms herself, but they are in very bard order now, and the ceiling is coming down. The first year after she moved in Trinity reduced the rent to $5, but the next year it was raised again to $5.50, and has remained at that ever since.

In one apartment on the top floor I found a tall, sickly looking man frying fish. A shapeless woman with an appealing look upon her face sat watching him.

He showed me the rooms, keeping a careful eye on the fish meanwhile, so that it might not burn. The walls in the bedroom were wet and the roof leaked in the other room.

The man told me that he used to be a boilermaker in the navy-yard, but his health failed and he was unable to work at his trade and was forced to do odd jobs when his health permitted. He has just returned from ten weeks spent in St. Vincent's Hospital.

I asked him what was wrong, and the shapeless woman in the chair answered for him.

"He's got the dropsy, poor dear," she said, the tears rolling over her cheeks, "an' they took twenty-six quarts of water from him in the hospital. I'm dying with the same thing. Look at my hands and legs! See, they ain't any shape to them. I sit here all the time waiting to die. I can't lie down in bed, 'cause I choke. An' I haven't a friend in the world.

I'm no kin of his, but him an' his wife took me in. They're good, and they deserve better luck than sickness.

I asked the man how they managed to exist, and he said his wife worked in Gordon & Dilworth's factory for seven cents an hour. She works ten hours a day, which means 70 cents, and would gladly work longer if her strength permitted.

The man told me also that when he moved in the rooms were so filthy that he had almost concluded not to take them, but the Trinity agents said if he would clean them himself they would allow him for it. But they have never done so, though he papered and whitewashed. They have even refused to pay for the lime.

On the same floor with him is a widow whose sole support is a boy who earns $5 a week in as cracker factory. The woman has "rheumatics so bad she can't touch the floor."

Her daughter, about fourteen years old, does the housework. The widow says she has lived there for fifteen years and has never owed Trinity until this month. She is back one dollar, and she sent her daughter out to pawn some clothes so she can pay that.

And this is only part of my experiences among the Trinity tenements.

Pictures of Nellie Bly

Nellie Bly,
Circa 1888

Nellie Bly, Circa
1890

Nellie Bly,
1890

Nellie Bly, Circa
1922

BOOK DEFINITIONS

1. Overkind: excessively and unnecessarily kind
2. Slavey: a female, domestic servant who does difficult physical work
3. Assentingly: to do something in an agreeable manner
4. Blasé': unconcerned or apathetic to pleasure
5. Quick: the connective tissue underneath the fingernail
6. Noddings: agreement or acceptance of something
7. Ablutions: washing, bathing; Can also be a house that contains bathing and toilet facilities
8. Aught: all, everything, anything
9. Passementerie: decorative, ornamental edging or trimming

ANNOTATIONS/BIOGRAPHY

Blackwell's Island Lunatic Asylum was established in 1834. And after construction, it opened in 1839. It was the very first asylum that was opened in New York, and later became a part of other lunatic asylums in New   York.

Due to overcrowding, conditions at the asylum were horrible. Overcrowding contributed to frequent disease outbreaks. Food was often spoiled, there were not enough employees to take care of patients, and prison inmates were often employed because of the scarcity of help at the asylum.

In the 1840's, Charles Dickens visited the asylum. After his visit Dickens wrote "...everything had a lounging, listless, madhouse air, which was very painful. The moping idiot, cowering down with long disheveled hair; the gibbering maniac, with his hideous laugh and pointed finger; the vacant eye, the fierce wild face, the gloomy picking of the hands and lips, and munching of the nails: there they were all, without disguise, in naked ugliness and horror."

In 1897, reporter Nellie Bly was admitted to the asylum in an attempt to do some undercover reporting on the conditions there. It was part of an assignment given to her by Joseph Pulitzer.   Nellie writes:

"What, excepting torture, would produce insanity quicker than this treatment? Here is a class of women sent to be cured. I would like the expert physicians who are condemning me for my action, which has proven their ability, to take a perfectly sane and healthy woman, shut her up and make her sit from 6 a.m. until 8 p.m. on straight-back benches, do not allow her to talk or move during these hours, give her no reading and let her know nothing of the world or its doings, give her bad food and harsh treatment, and see how long it will take to make her insane. Two months would make her a mental and physical wreck."

She also wrote: "The insane asylum on Blackwell's Island is a human rat-trap. It is easy to get in, but once there it is impossible to get out."

While in the asylum, Bly was witness to beatings, neglect, rotten food, very poor living conditions and many more atrocities.   She had the opportunity to observe and talk with many women, some of whom didn't appear to be insane. Some women did not speak English as a first language and were in the asylum merely because they couldn't communicate well with others who spoke English. Other women were in the asylum under different circumstances, but also did not appear to be insane.

Joseph Pulitzer got her released after 10 days of her being there.

Due to Bly's book, <u>Ten Days in A Mad-House</u>, the Blackwell's Island Lunatic Aslum was given $1 million in funds, and shortly closed thereafter in April 1894.

The author of this book, Nellie Bly, was also known as Elizabeth Cochran Seaman. She was an American journalist, who wrote <u>Ten Days in A Mad-House</u>, <u>Around the World In 72</u> Days and <u>Six Months in Mexico</u>.

Nellie Bly was born May 5, 1864 and died of pneumonia at the age of 57 in 1922.

Notes

Notes

Notes

Made in the USA
Monee, IL
15 October 2021